Col

5-m Stress-busting

/icky Hales-Dutton

First published in 2007 by Collins, an imprint of HarperCollins *Publishers*
77–85 Fulham Palace Road, Hammersmith, London W6 8JB
everything clicks: www.collins.co.uk

Created by: **Focus Publishing**, Sevenoaks, Kent
Editor: Guy Croton
Designer/Illustrator: Diarmuid Moloney
Project co-ordinator: Caroline Watson

A catalogue record for this book is available from the British Library

ISBN–10: 00 00 724387 1
ISBN–13: 978 0 00 724387 7

This book is proudly printed on paper which contains wood from well managed forests, certified in accordance with the rules of the Forest Stewardship Council.
For more information about FSC,
please visit www.fsc-uk.org

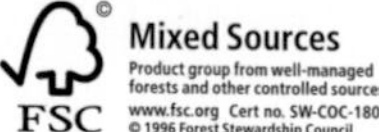

Printed and bound by Amadeus

CONTENTS

INTRODUCTION

SO YOU ARE FEELING STRESSED?

If feeling tense,'sick with worry', or overwhelmed with work is familiar territory for you, then you know what it's like to suffer with stress. Perhaps you've suffered from physical symptoms, like a persistent headache or dry mouth? Most of us struggle at times to cope with the ups and downs of daily life, and this is normal. But when stress continues over a long period, or you're dealing with life-changing events such as moving house or coping with bereavement, you need to know how to minimize your stress levels. The most important thing to remember is that you're not alone. Our fast pace of life, and the pressure to look good and be successful in everything we do, means stress is more prevalent than ever. A survey commissioned by the Samaritans found that 59% of people in the UK said they felt 'stressed out' at least once a month. Work is partly to blame.

An international problem

According to the International Stress Management Association, 70% of adults are stressed at work. That translates into the loss of 13 million working days each year to stress, costing UK organizations £4 billion.

Although it's difficult to draw like-for-like comparisons with other countries because their measurement of data can differ markedly, we do know that stress, particularly work-related stress, is an international problem.

A study entitled 'Work and Health in the EU – A Statistical Portrait', shows that in1999 more UK people (especially women) reported work-related stress, depression and anxiety than their European colleagues. Portugal came second, with Spanish workers the least stressed. Across the Atlantic, a 1997 survey by Yale University showed that 29% of American workers felt 'quite a bit' or 'extremely' stressed.

Long hours

The long hours culture doesn't help. In 2002 a survey found that the UK worked the longest hours in Europe – over 43 per week, with 10 per cent of employees clocking up a 61-hour week – and took the shortest holidays, with just 20 days annual leave. This compares with Europe's 40-hour average working week and holidays as long as 38 days in, for example, Austria.

What is stress?

The Health & Safety Executive defines stress as 'the adverse reaction people have to excessive pressure or other types of demand placed on them'. Dr Chris

Johnstone, author of *Find Your Power*, describes it as 'an imbalance where the demands experienced by someone exceed what they can happily cope with'.

Experts agree that some pressure can be useful, spurring us on to greater achievements so we can reach our full potential. But when the pressure is too great – and this varies from person to person – the body cannot cope and starts to display a variety of physical and mental symptoms. This is when 'normal' everyday pressure ends and stress begins.

The stress response is first and foremost a survival mechanism. The human body responds instinctively to danger by preparing physically and mentally for either 'fight or flight' – doing battle or running away very fast!

Fight or flight

When we are under threat our bodies release a variety of chemical messengers and hormones such as adrenaline, noradrenaline and cortisol. These act rapidly – oxygen is pumped faster round our bodies and our brains and muscles get a bumper supply of blood, diverted from other areas such as digestion – so that we can think and act quickly. This undoubtedly served our ancestors well in deciding whether to fight the sabre-toothed tiger or run away from it, and the physical exertion in either activity would have neutralized the effects of the chemicals and hormones in their bodies.

Our everyday worries are different now. While not immediately life-threatening, traffic jams and money problems still trigger the same chemical response as that hungry sabre-toothed tiger did all those millennia ago.

We take less exercise nowadays, so the body retains those chemicals and hormones which, admittedly, help to boost our performance in the short term. However, it's when our worries persist and there is no physical outlet that stress becomes harmful.

What can we do about it?

Recognizing that a problem exists can be difficult. By reading this book you have taken the first step on your journey towards combating stress!

There's no single, magic solution. What works for one person may not work for another. So we've included some tried and tested stress-busting techniques, practical hints and tips. Try these, even if you don't believe they'll make a difference. You could be pleasantly surprised at how much better you feel, and how quickly, too! It's your life, remember, and there's no reason why you shouldn't spend some quality time on you – for a change.

WHAT IS STRESS?

This chapter examines the causes of stress, its physical, mental and emotional effects and the potential impact it has on how people behave.

THE NERVOUS SYSTEM

Let's begin with a look at the physiological origins of the stress – or 'fight or flight' – response, which is the responsibility of the body's autonomic nervous system.

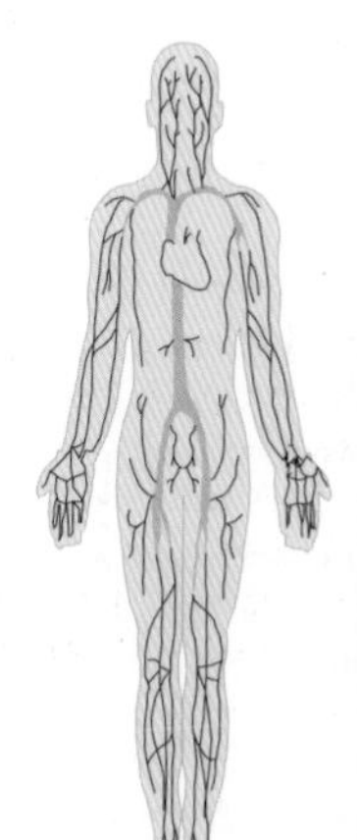

The body's network of nerve cells carry rapid messages from one part to another – about what's happening inside the body or about the outside world. The human nervous system is made up of several interconnected parts, including:

The central nervous system.

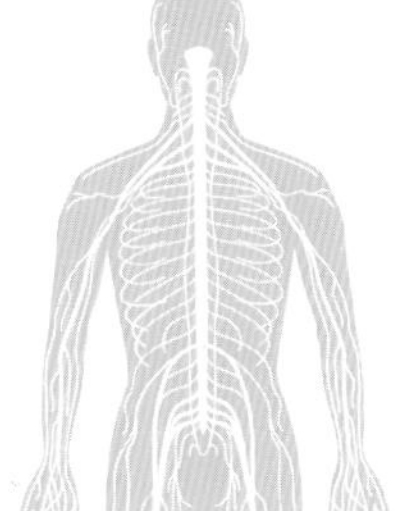

The autonomic nervous system.

1) The **central nervous system** – comprising the brain and spinal chord, this integrates the body's entire nervous function.
2) The **peripheral nervous system** – its nerves gather information or transmit orders.
3) The **somatic nervous system** – its nerves send information to the brain relating to the external environment gained via the senses.
4) The **autonomic nervous system** – its nerves regulate the body's internal organs, co-ordinating activities like breathing, heart rate, circulation, hormone secretion, perspiration and digestion. The autonomic nervous system is divided into the sympathetic and parasympathetic nervous systems. The **sympathetic** nervous system readies the body for action. The **parasympathetic** nervous system slows down and reduces what has been accelerated or triggered via the sympathetic nervous system, shutting off the body's fight or flight reaction so you can relax. This is what happens when you become stressed....

THE STRESS CYCLE

When people are afraid or under pressure the brain's hypothalamus sends signals (via the pituitary gland) to the adrenal glands (on the kidneys). These release the hormones adrenaline, noradrenaline and cortisol into the bloodstream.

The hypothalamus is situated (with the pituitary gland) at the base of the brain. It is responsible for the overall co-ordination of hormone secretion. The adrenal gland – an endocrine gland situated on top of the kidney – plays a major role in the body's short-term stress response. Its outer part (cortex) secretes hormones like cortisol, which regulates the use of carbohydrates, proteins, and fats and shuts down the immune system. Its inner section (medulla) secretes the hormones adrenaline and noradrenalin – the 'fight or flight' chemicals.

Hormones are neurotransmitters or chemical messengers that affect certain organs. The stress hormones cortisol, adrenaline and noradrenaline impact on the major organs in different ways. Long-term stress can affect the adrenals themselves. Persistent overwork because of the constant requirement for stress hormones can lead to fatigue and depression. The adrenals can eventually shut down.

gan	What happens when you're stressed
n	Increased blood supply and energy from the release of sugars. 'Non-essential' functions like memory and concentration are switched off.
uth	Less saliva.
cles	Increased blood supply, tense and ready for action.
rt/circulation	Increased heart rate/blood pressure.
gs	Increased respiration, faster breathing (from the top of the chest).
nach	Reduced blood supply, more acid secretion ('butterflies' in stomach).
dder	Frequent urination due to stimulated nervous system.
s	Pupils dilate.
stines (including colon)	Reduced blood supply.
estive contractions	Speed up or slow down, leading to diarrhoea or constipation.
n	Reduced blood supply and increased perspiration
neral biochemistry	Increased energy and higher consumption of fats and sugars
nune system	Deemed non-essential so shuts down

A VICIOUS CIRCLE

Stress can seriously affect the mind and the body, sometimes separately and often at the same time. It can have a dramatic effect on the way people behave which can profoundly – and negatively – influence their lives for years if nothing is done about it.

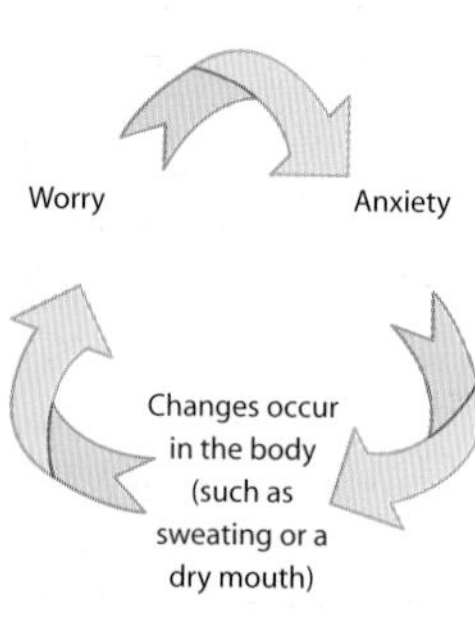

The vicious circle that is stress. The more problems persist, the worse they get.

People faced with emotionally demanding situations over a long period can reach 'burnout' – physical, mental and emotional exhaustion. The sufferer experiences feelings of hopelessness, disillusionment and cynicism (plus the usual physical, mental and emotional symptoms of stress).

Negative behaviours can take on a life of their own. If you're prone to anxiety, for example, the thought pattern probably looks a bit like the diagram above. You need to break this cycle so that you can cope better with your stress and start living life to the full.

Nowadays people rarely face acute physical danger but the body's response to fear, anger or upset remains the same. At their desks or in their cars, though, there are few opportunities for physical activity to shut down the stress cycle, stop the flow of hormones (which can take just half an hour to release and several days to expel from the body) and bring them back into equilibrium.

Physical and mental stress-related illnesses are a response to the constant flow of stress hormones. These illnesses are stressful in themselves, and so begins a vicious circle. Breaking free means understanding the changes that occur during a stress reaction and allowing the body to do its vital job of restoring the balance.

Recognizing those early warning signs

Sooner or later, too much strain takes its toll and various physical and/or mental symptoms appear. Initially these can occur in existing weak spots. So, for example, if you have a sensitive digestion, watch out for stomach upsets and nausea. It's not always easy to make the link between these initial symptoms and stress. But they're usually the first indication that something is wrong, so now is the time to take action to prevent the problem from getting out of hand. Although everyone's bodies are different, the symptoms listed on the following page are common early warning signs of stress overload.

Early warning physical symptoms

Nausea – possibly the most common physical symptom of stress.

Indigestion – often a sharp pain in the centre of the chest and occurring soon after eating.

Headaches – are a good indication of stress. Tension headaches are usually caused by sustained contraction of the scalp, face and neck muscles, resulting in a painful throbbing affecting any part of the head.

Dry mouth – stress causes saliva to cease flowing, causing a dry mouth.

Persistent diarrhoea (frequent passing of liquid stools) for over three days. If the nerve endings in the 9m long gastro-intestinal tract become over-stimulated and the bowel muscles are tense, colonic contractions can get more intense and the pressure build-up can result in diarrhoea.

Sleeping difficulties, including insomnia – sufferers either cannot get to sleep or they wake up frequently, and their sleep is of poor quality.
(See Chapter 7.)

Palpitations (a rapidly beating heart) – on average the normal human heart beats about once a second, but physical and mental exertion can cause it to beat faster temporarily. If your palpitations are accompanied by pain and shortness of breath, see your GP immediately.

Early warning mental symptoms

Over-reacting to little things – burning the toast could be the straw that breaks the camel's back.

Impulsive behaviour. You do things without thinking through the consequences.

Inability to concentrate on anything for more than a few minutes.

Irritability and short temper. You snap at people for no reason.

LONGER-TERM SYMPTOMS OF STRESS

Over the longer term, people who feel stressed may well experience a wide variety of other physical and emotional symptoms that can become established, resulting in noticeable behavioural changes.These symptoms can also indicate problems other than stress, so check with your GP if in doubt.

Longer term physical symptoms

Condition	Characterized by
Allergies	Including hay fever.
Asthma and shortness of breath	Coughing.
Digestive problems	Bloating, burning, cramping, irritable bowel syndrome, peptic ulcers.
Eating patterns	Loss of appetite (and weight), craving 'comfort foods', causing weight gain.
Menstrual difficulties	Irregular, painful or scanty periods.
Migraine	A headache lasting between 4–72 hours, often with nausea and visual disturbances.
Pain caused by muscle tension	Especially in the back, shoulders and neck.
Pins and needles in the fingers	Caused by heightened nerve sensitivity.

(continued overleaf)

Skin problems	Unexplained itching, worsening of eczema, psoriasis and acne.
Susceptibility to infections	Less effective immune system, longer recovery time after illness.
Sexual problems	Reduced fertility, temporary impotence (men) difficulty in achieving orgasm (women).
Tiredness	Usually caused by lack of good quality, refreshing sleep as your sleeping patterns change.

Longer term mental symptoms

Condition	Characterized by
Anxious feelings	See opposite.
Depressed feelings	Feeling 'overwhelmed' can lead to a lack of energy and the will to do anything. If left untreated, eating or sleeping disorders can occur.
Feeling unable to cope	Everyday tasks seem overwhelming.
Low self esteem	Feeling worthless, your confidence plummets.
Mood swings	Feeling positive one minute, low the next.
Poor short-term memory	Stress affects the parts of the brain governing short-term memory and concentration.
Irrational thought	You over-react and behave out of character.

Anxious feelings

These occur because of the body's immediate reaction to stress. According to the mental health charity Mind, 1 in 20 people suffer with an anxiety disorder at any one time. Anxiety can occur as a result of:

- Concern about something that will happen, like a job interview or life changing event.
- Blowing something out of proportion, giving it sinister qualities that it doesn't have.
- Anticipating a situation that's never likely to occur.
- Not having enough information about something.
- Having too much information. This leads to panic because you can't process and understand it all.

Often, the more anxious you feel, the more you worry about feeling anxious, and physical symptoms of anxiety, such as a racing heart, sweating, tight chest or shallow breathing, can become frightening, which establishes a vicious circle.

Most people feel anxious sometimes, especially before a job interview, an exam, or similar. In fact, the adrenaline can help enhance your performance and bring you up to the task in hand. This situational anxiety normally settles fairly quickly. However, if it persists over a period of time, seek medical help.

The following can occur when people are stressed:

Emotional/behavioural symptoms

Condition	Characterized by
Bullying	Shouting,being angry/abusive at home/work.
Edginess	Racing thoughts and constant worrying.
Hostility	You resent colleagues or customers.
Inability to relax	Restlessness and constant activity.
Increased drinking/smoking	Weight gain/liver/chest problems.
Loss of libido/performance	More anxiety, less confidence.
Noise intolerance	Sudden loud noises seem unbearable.
Poor time management	Unable to complete tasks on time, or at all.
Thinking about harming self/others	Maybe leading to suicide/violence.
Uncontrollable emotions	Crying at the slightest provocation.
Worries about one's health	Leading to anxiety/physical symptoms.

HOW STRESSED ARE YOU?

It's time to see how stress is affecting you, your body and your life. The following questionnaires are designed to gauge how stressed you are, which are the problem areas in your life and how good your support network is.

You and your body questionnaire

Let's start with any physical and mental symptoms you may have. Put a tick next to each symptom you now have, count these up and check your score on page 21.

Physical symptoms

Allergies, including hay fever		Dry mouth	
Asthma/coughing		Headaches	
Change in eating patterns:		High blood pressure	
• food cravings/weight gain		Migraine	
• loss of appetite (and weight)		Back, shoulder, neck pain	
Chest pain and/or palpitations		Pins and needles (fingers)	
		Skin problems	
Digestive problems		Sleep problems/tiredness	
• nausea		Susceptibility to infections	
• constipation		Sexual problems:	
• cramping		• problems achieving orgasm	
• diarrhoea		• reduced fertility	
• indigestion		• temporary impotence	

Emotional symptoms – Behavioural symptoms

Emotional symptoms		Behavioural symptoms	
Anxious feelings		Accident prone	
Considers harming others		Attempted suicide	
Considers harming self		Bullying	
Depressed feelings		Cannot express feelings	
Feeling angry		Cannot relax	
Feeling disillusioned		Changes in sleeping	
Feeling guilty		Cynical behaviour	
Feeling helpless/ defenceless		Distant from family/friends	
		Edginess	
Feeling out of control		Flagging work performance	
Feelings of hopelessness		Hostility	
Feelings of shame		Hurts others	
Feeling unable to cope		Hurts self	
Feeling uneasy		Impulsive behaviour	
Imagination working overtime		Irritability	
		More drinking/smoking	
Lack of confidence/ self esteem		Loss of appetite	
		Loss of interest in sex	
Lack of enthusiasm		Mood swings	
Loss of confidence in own judgement		Noise intolerance	
		Overeating	
Worries about own health		Poor concentration	
Worries about the health of others		Poor judgement	
		Poor short-term memory	
Uncontrollable emotions		Poor time management	

Negative thoughts

Put a tick next to each thought you have regularly now:

'I should cope better'

'Everyone's against me'

'I can't do simple tasks any more'

'No-one understands me'

'I'll never be able to do it'

'What's the use in trying?'

'I wish I were dead'

'I've lost confidence in making good decisions'

'I feel overwhelmed'

'I don't know what to do'

I'm so forgetful'

'I worry about everything'

I'm a failure'

'No-one cares'

'I can't do it'

'There's no point in anything'

Your body's stress rating

0–4 symptoms – You have few symptoms and are probably not too stressed now. But watch out for any future symptoms. The questionnaires on pages 22–8 should provide some useful clues.

10–14 symptoms – You're moderately stressed and should make changes to your life now. Try the questionnaires on pages 22–8.

15 or more symptoms – You're very stressed and should take immediate action to tackle this. The questionnaires on pages 22–8 will help.

Next, I'd like you to take a closer look at your relationships with family and friends and leisure activities.

Family relationships	Yes	No
Do you have a close, loving, open and honest relationship with your partner?		
Do you make an effort in the relationship, even when things are not going well?		
Do you listen to his/her problems and help him/her work through them?		
If you both work, do you share household chores and childcare equally?		
Do you spend adequate time with family?		
Do you feel loved and valued?		
Are you close to your children?		

Friendships	Yes	No
Are friends important to you?		
Do you have a small circle of close friends?		
Do you prefer a large circle of acquaintances?		
Do friends provide help and support?		
Do you offer help/support to friends?		
Do you see friends regularly?		
Do you actively keep in touch with them?		
Can you say no to friends?		
Can you trust them not to take advantage?		
Can you trust friends with confidences?		

Leisure time

Leisure time	Yes	No
Do you enjoy the time you spend with family?		
Do you have a regular hobby?		
Do you take plenty of exercise?		
Can you escape from email/mobile phones for at least part of your weekend/holiday?		
Do you enjoy a bit of healthy competition?		
Do you take at least one family holiday a year?		
Do you regularly do activities together as a family?		

Your score

If you answered mainly **'yes'** throughout this questionnaire, your life generally seems solid. Don't worry about a few 'nos' – no-one's life is perfect after all! Focus on one problem area at a time and tackle it by breaking it down into more easily-manageable chunks.

If your **'no'** answers outnumbered the 'yes' answers, look at the most urgent area first. Try breaking this down so that you're able to complete each task, bit by bit. Look at the easier areas first – seeing positive results quickly will boost your confidence.

This book will show you a number of techniques that will help you manage your stess – and change in one area may positively affect the others!

Stress at work questionnaire

Is your workplace stressful? Find out by circling whichever number applies in each question and adding up your score:

	Never	Rarely	Sometimes	Often	Always
'My boss is supportive'	1	2	3	4	5
'I get on with colleagues'	1	2	3	4	5
'There's time to do my work'	1	2	3	4	5
'I have the equipment & resources to do the job'	1	2	3	4	5
'I feel recognized, valued & rewarded'	1	2	3	4	5
'Feedback is constructive'	1	2	3	4	5
'There are promotion opportunities'	1	2	3	4	5
'I can take time off for family problems'	1	2	3	4	5
'I always leave promptly'	1	2	3	4	5
'Action is taken against office bullies'	1	2	3	4	5
'I am adequately trained'	1	2	3	4	5
'I take my full holiday'	1	2	3	4	5
'There's enough work'	1	2	3	4	5
'I love going to work'	1	2	3	4	5
'I don't take work home'	1	2	3	4	5

Your score

15–30 points – Your work stress levels are extremely high. You're overworked and don't feel supported or valued. Can you talk to anyone in confidence – your boss, their boss, a colleague, your human resources department? This isn't just your problem, it's your organization's too – and it should take responsibility.

31–45 points – Your workplace is stressful. Look again at the problem areas and see how you can tackle these, preferably one at a time! Try talking to your boss or someone else at work to see if they can help or advise you.

46–60 points – Your organization is generally supportive and you can work without undue stress. If there are busy periods, try to plan for those in advance. Can you do anything during quiet times that would lift the load during the busy ones?

61–75 points – You clearly work in a super environment. There may be few obvious causes of stress now, but things can change and it's a good idea to be aware of what triggers stress in you.

HOW STRESSFUL IS YOUR LIFE?

However big or small, any change to our lives can be stressful, even positive ones like getting married. In the quiz on the following page by American psychologists Holmes & Rahe, each event is scored into Life Change Units, according to their degree of stress.

Life change questionnaire

If you've experienced any of the following within the last two years, tick the relevant box and add up your score.

Event	Scale	You
Death of a partner	100	
Divorce	75	
Separation from partner	65	
Jail sentence	63	
Death of a close family member	63	
Personal injury or illness	53	
Marriage	50	
Loss of job	47	
Reconciliation with a partner	45	
Retirement	45	
Change in your/family's health	44	
Pregnancy	40	
Sexual difficulties	39	
New family member	39	
Major business or work changes	39	
Change in your financial state	38	
Death of close friend	37	
Arguments with a partner	36	
Large mortgage	31	
Foreclosure of a mortgage or loan	30	
Change in responsibilities at work	29	
Son or daughter leaving home	29	

Event	Scale	You
Trouble with in-laws	29	
Outstanding personal achievement	28	
Partner begins or stops work	26	
Child begins or finishes school	26	
Change in living conditions	25	
Change in personal habits	24	
Trouble with boss	23	
Change in working hours/conditions	20	
Change in residence	19	
Change of school	19	
Change in social activities	18	
Low mortgage or loan	17	
Change in sleeping habits	16	
Change in number of family gatherings	15	
Change in eating habits	15	
Going on holiday	13	
Christmas	12	
Minor violations of the law	11	
Your total		

Your score

Over 300 points – You're very stressed and risk developing a serious stress-related illness. You must take steps now to lower your stress level.

200–299 points – You're under pressure, and must reduce your stress levels.

150–200 points – This is mild to moderate, but some changes are needed.

Under 150 points – This is reasonable, but always keep an eye on it.

HOW SUPPORTED ARE YOU?

Who do you turn to when you're most in need? Find out by trying the quick quiz below. For each question, circle a number on a scale between 0–5, where 0 equates to No and 5 is Yes.

	No					Yes
'I have several friends/family members with whom I can talk openly about problems/feelings'	0	1	2	3	4	5
'I have friends on whom I can call at any time'	0	1	2	3	4	5
'I spend time with people I like and respect, rather than just acquaintances and colleagues'	0	1	2	3	4	5
'People look for my friendship'	0	1	3	3	4	5

Your score

Mostly 4 and 5 – You have a super support network. But it cuts both ways – others need your support sometimes, too.

Mostly 3 – This could be better. Try confiding in friends and family more often and asking for help when you need it.

Mostly 0–2 – You have little support. Do you help others when they need it? Surround yourself with those you can rely on.

KNOW YOURSELF:
The role of personality

Many psychologists say that what makes people feel stressed, by how much and how they cope is closely linked to their personality.

Everyone is different when it comes to how much pressure they can bear before it becomes too much. Someone with a low stress threshold can become anxious about losing their TV remote control or being slightly late for work, for example. Others may take these minor irritations in their stride but worry about moving house or making a presentation at work.

The experts have different theories about how people's personalities are formed – and rarely agree with one another! Some believe that personality is developed in early childhood and we learn by what our parents do. So, if they remain cool under pressure, we are likely to behave in the same way.

Some theories say genes are more influential than environment. So certain personalities are more prone to stress-related illnesses because of their genetic make-up. Other studies show that it's down to a child's experience in the womb, with stressed pregnant women more likely to give birth to children with emotional difficulties.

Type A vs Type B

Psychologists classify human behaviour in various ways, but one simple method is to divide people into Type A or Type B personalities. Which are you? Find out by trying the quick quiz below. Tick x or y, whichever applies:

x

- Casual about being on time
- Slow and relaxed
- Not worried about about deadlines
- Not very competitive
- Not overly ambitious
- Listens well
- Feels there's lots of time
- Can wait patiently
- Does one task at a time
- Speaks more slowly
- Seeks recognition
- Is easy-going
- Likes to be busy but not frantic
- Can express feelings freely
- Has lots of hobbies

y

- Worries about being late but often is!
- Has few interests outside school/work
- Keen to get things done
- Very competitive
- Very ambitious
- A poor listener
- Always in a rush
- Hates waiting
- Does several things at once
- Speaks quickly/forcefully
- Seeks a hectic lifestyle
- Pushes self and others hard
- Hides feelings
- Does everything quickly
- Doesn't care what others think

How you scored:
Mostly x – You're a Type B personality.
Mostly y – You're a Type A personality.

Because it's a sliding scale, most people will incline towards Type A or Type B, rather than being totally one or the other. But the closer you are to a particular type, the more likely you will display characteristics associated with that personality.

Type As do everything quickly, they're competitive and often perfectionists. They're less able to take life's ups and downs in their stride, finding even small disruptions to their routine upsetting. They are more prone to stress. Type Bs are more easy-going and adaptable. They are able to put things into perspective and can therefore cope better with what life throws at them.

Type As are more likely to suffer with stress-related illnesses like high blood pressure or to overindulge in alcohol or cigarettes. Studies have also shown that anger or hostility – a typical Type A behavioural trait – can increase the risk of raised blood pressure, doubling the likelihood of heart attacks in susceptible people.

Type A personalities really need to develop techniques for reducing stress. This book will show you how this is done!

THE GENDER GAP

The way people deal with stress is also linked to gender. Experts say that men and women get upset by different things – and react in different ways. Nowadays most women have a job, and so face workplace pressures in addition to household chores and looking after children. Balancing the needs of their home and working lives can be stressful, especially if these two worlds collide, for example, when their families are ill.

Fortunately many (although by no means all) women are 'multi-tasked' – they can do several things at once, which helps them cope with life's many demands.

Things have changed for men, too, in recent years. Long hours, the relentless march of technology and the spectre of long-term unemployment (which is greater for men) have all piled on the pressure. They're also expected to be perfect partners and fathers, so it is not surprising that men have become vulnerable to stress.

Whereas women are happier to seek medical help, men often only visit their GP when they get the physical symptoms of stress, like chest pains or headaches, while depression can often go undiagnosed.

For example, men are more likely than women to repress their feelings, escape via drink or drugs, use violence, drive recklessly, be depressed – and even to commit suicide.

How do you cope with problems?

As you've seen, different personalities deal with what life throws at them in different ways. Most people resort to tried and tested ways of dealing with life's problems, whether or not these offer a long-term solution. Find out your preferred method with the following quiz:

A work colleague gets the promotion you've been expecting. How do you react? Tick the box that applies to you.

1) You blame your manager.
2) You weren't meant to get it. Anyway, others would be resentful and you don't need the extra money.
3) You escape into your own world where you're the boss and the new appointee reports to you.
4) You're upset but you shake it off – and think about how well you'll do in the forthcoming local squash club's championships.
5) You don't care. There's no point in trying so you might as well give up on promotion right now.
6) You kick the cat (or anything else in your way).
7) You get very drunk.

How did you score?

If you ticked **(1)** you're projecting your feelings onto someone or something else. You need someone to blame for not getting the job, because it is too painful to accept that you didn't have the right skills, attitude or whatever else the boss was looking for. Next time, be honest about what went wrong and you'll learn for next time. Breaking out of this pattern may be stressful at first but will reap rewards in the long run.

If you ticked **(2)** you use rationalization to console yourself. You tell yourself that you're not upset because you didn't expect to get the promotion anyway, and you've actually had a lucky escape. Rationalization can be a cosy cocoon, but beware the partner or friend who points out the truth – that you wouldn't have gone for the promotion in the first place if you didn't actually want it!

If you ticked **(3)** you're an escape artist, regularly slipping into a comfortable day-dream to block out sad and hurtful things. Do try to keep a grip on what's real and what isn't, or you could be in for a bumpy ride!

Did you choose **(4)**? Then you are compensating for not getting promoted by focusing on success in another area. There's nothing wrong with that but be aware of how you are feeling and why. It can be easy to over-compensate for disappointment, which can result in a state of denial.

Ticking **(5)** means that apathy is your chosen way of dealing with life. Sometimes problems can disappear if we ignore them but often they get worse, not better. Facing up to them isn't easy, but burying one's head in the sand could turn a little problem into a really big one.

If you ticked **(6)** you're displaying displaced aggression. You have no physical outlet for your anger so you take it out on someone or something else. Try to get out of this habit. It's distressing for others and your relationships could suffer. The best way to deal with anger is to do something physical – a vigorous game of squash, an aerobics class or lifting some weights will all help.

If **(7)** is your preferred method and you regularly over-indulge in food, alcohol, cigarettes or drugs, you could have a dependency or an eating disorder. If so, you may need medical help.

Later in this book you will be exploring other, more constructive ways of dealing with problems.

THE STORY SO FAR...

Hopefully after reading this chapter and working through the stress questionnaires, you now understand more about stress and the role it plays in your life. However, before moving onto Chapter 2, let's pause for one final exercise. Jot your answers to the following questions (and any other thoughts) on some paper:

- List three things that most annoy or depress you. What can you do about these?

- List the things you expect yourself to do (for example, cleaning the house each day, always preparing home-made cakes or packed lunches for your partner/teenage children, driving family and friends short distances when they could walk). What would happen if you didn't do each one? Who would benefit/suffer or even notice? To restore balance, something may need to go, so decide which one it is.

- Now I'd like you to consider your needs. On one side of the page list everything that you find draining about your life. On the other side list the things in life that regularly fulfil you and keep you feeling happy. How does the balance look?

- Do you have clear goals and have you achieved any, or are they just pipedreams?

Keep your answers to these questions in a safe place. You'll probably refer to them again when you reach Chapter 8, 'Longer Term Solutions'.

Let's move on to Chapter 2.

LEARNING TO RELAX

WHAT IS RELAXATION?

Rest, refreshment, recreation, chilling out, switching off, taking five and hanging loose are all words associated with relaxation. Or, put another way, taking a break from an activity that requires concentration or hard physical effort, and doing something enjoyable – or nothing at all!

Relaxation involves giving yourself time and space to recover physically and mentally from situations that cause stress and anxiety.

When people feel threatened they often resort to the fight or flight response. But their bodies strive for equilibrium and try to recover when the danger diminishes. So often, though, the body is not allowed to do its job. You may be exhausted but you keep pushing yourself harder– and wonder why you feel ill. It's hardly surprising that many people no longer know how to switch off.

But all is not lost! Even five minutes' relaxation each day can make a difference to how you'll feel and behave. The rest of this chapter aims to help you understand why relaxation matters – and, more importantly, how you can learn to relax properly and begin reaping the benefits.

ARE YOU ABLE TO RELAX?

How well can you relax? Circle whichever number applies to you in each question and add up your score.

	Never	Rarely	Sometimes	Often	Always
'I take on too much'	1	2	3	4	5
'I can't sit still'	1	2	3	4	5
'I rarely finish anything'	1	2	3	4	5
'I can't concentrate on a TV or radio programme'	1	2	3	4	5
'My muscles are tense'	1	2	3	4	5
'I clench my jaw and/or grind my teeth'	1	2	3	4	5
'My thoughts flit about'	1	2	3	4	5
'I suffer from panic attacks'	1	2	3	4	5
'Everyone else is doing better'	1	2	3	4	5
'I eat my meals on the go'	1	2	3	4	5
'I don't take my full holiday entitlement'	1	2	3	4	5
'I feel I don't have any fun'	1	2	3	4	5
'I snack on fast foods and carbonated drinks'	1	2	3	4	5
'I worry about getting everything done'	1	2	3	4	5
'I skip breakfast'	1	2	3	4	5
'I have problems sleeping'	1	2	3	4	5
'I get indigestion after meals'	1	2	3	4	5

	Never	Rarely	Sometimes	Often	Always
'I rush, even on holiday'	1	2	3	4	5
'I neglect my hobbies'	1	2	3	4	5
'I neglect family and friends'	1	2	3	4	5
'I take my laptop or mobile phone on holiday'	1	3	4	4	5
'I feel anxious'	1	2	3	4	5
'It's difficult to switch off'	1	2	3	4	5
'I worry something terrible will happen'	1	2	3	4	5
'No-one listens to my worries'	1	2	3	4	5
'I skip exercise'	1	2	3	4	5
'I have caffeinated drinks'	1	2	3	4	5
'I have sugary food several times a day'	1	2	3	4	5
'I work more than 40 hours a week'	1	2	3	4	5
'I take work home'	1	2	3	4	5
'It's difficult to communicate with my partner/family'	1	2	3	4	5
'There's no time to play with my children'	1	2	3	4	5
'There's no time to listen'	1	2	3	4	5
'I fix back-to-back meetings'	1	2	3	4	5
'I sleep for less than 7 hours'	1	2	3	4	5
'I rush through meals'	1	2	3	4	5
'I argue with my partner/family'	1	2	3	4	5

	Never	Rarely	Sometimes	Often	Always
'I regularly suffer with constipation or diarrhoea'	1	2	3	4	5
'Other drivers annoy me'	1	2	3	4	5
'I smoke more than ten cigarettes a day'	1	2	3	4	5
'I work late two evenings or more per week'	1	2	3	4	5
'I'm always competitive'	1	2	3	4	5
'I hunch over my computer'	1	2	3	4	5

Your score

Mostly 1s and 2s –You're generally able to relax. But tension can creep in and become established before you realize it. It's a good idea to do the quiz regularly – say every three months – to check you're keeping on top of it all.

Mostly 3s and 4s – You can relax at times but pressure affects your ability to switch off. You must address this, or your stress levels will continue to creep up and you will forget how to relax.

Mostly 5s and 6s – For you, relaxation is something you dream of doing but never do. Stress hormones are flowing all the time and you're in danger of a stress-related physical and mental illness. Please take action now to reduce your stress levels.

The quiz looked at four aspects of your life – work, eating/sleeping healthily, relationships and leisure. If any are a problem, break them into manageable chunks. Learning some relaxation techniques will help you through this and will soon enable you to regain a feeling of control.

HOW RELAXATION AFFECTS THE MIND AND BODY

The link between the mind and body is well documented and everyone now recognizes that the state of one affects the other. We know that mental pressure, stress and anxiety cause the physical symptoms that we discussed in Chapter 1. The immune system is also affected, and so persistent, long-term stress can result in serious illness.

The good news is that relaxation does the opposite. It stops the flow of stress hormones and strengthens the immune system. Studies have also shown that people who laugh more are generally fitter and healthier than those who don't, which just proves that laughter really is the best medicine. Have you ever noticed how much better a good laugh can make you feel?

Allowing yourself to recover from intense physical and mental effort by doing something you enjoy, such as participating in sport, learning a musical instrument or playing with your children, will make you feel good. So does doing absolutely nothing at all, because it gives you time and space for recuperation. The table opposite gives some examples of how both body and mind can benefit from being more relaxed (although these are symptoms are unrelated to each other).

Body	Mind
Heart stops racing	Less anxious
Regular, deeper breathing	More positive
Less muscle tension	Better able to face the day
Better digestion	See things in perspective
Fewer sexual problems	Think more clearly
Less susceptible to illness	More in control
More energy	Can deal better with stress
Sleep better	Enoy life more

The human muscle system

Each human body contains many muscles that hold it together, and allow for co-ordinated movement. These are attached to bones via connective tissue called tendons. So, whenever you move, the muscles contract and pull against those bones. Muscles work in pairs – and in opposite directions – so as one contracts (becomes shorter), pulling against a bone, the opposing muscle stretches to allow the movement. If muscles are taut or contracted, it's impossible for them to relax. A relaxed muscle feels soft, whereas a contracted muscle is much firmer. In between being contracted and being stretched there is the 'position of ease' – when your arm hangs loosely or your hand is not clenched but is soft and open. It's only when all your muscles are in the position of ease that you can be truly relaxed.

BODY AWARENESS

Are your muscles relaxed or taut? How much physical tension do you have in your body? If you answer 'yes' to any of the questions in the diagram below, then you clearly have some physical tension that needs to be addressed.

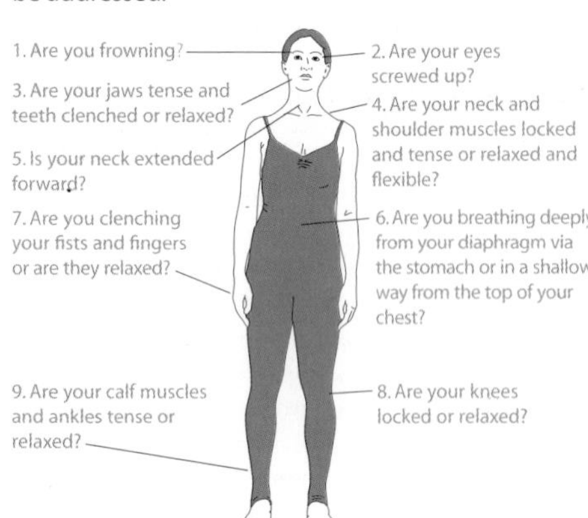
1. Are you frowning?
2. Are your eyes screwed up?
3. Are your jaws tense and teeth clenched or relaxed?
4. Are your neck and shoulder muscles locked and tense or relaxed and flexible?
5. Is your neck extended forward?
6. Are you breathing deeply from your diaphragm via the stomach or in a shallow way from the top of your chest?
7. Are you clenching your fists and fingers or are they relaxed?
8. Are your knees locked or relaxed?
9. Are your calf muscles and ankles tense or relaxed?

Start relaxing now!

Let's get on with some relaxation. When you first start, choose a quiet place where you won't be interrupted. Eventually, though, you'll be able relax anywhere.
Try this simple exercise first:

CANDLE FLAME RELAXATION

This involves focusing the mind on a specific object – the flame of a candle.

1) Darken the room.
2) Light a candle.
3) Get comfortable.
4) Gaze at the flame.
5) If your mind wanders, bring your focus back to the flame.
6) Do this for as long as you wish.
7) Extinguish the flame safely after use.

Does your mind feel calmer now? If so, then your body probably will, too.

PROGRESSIVE MUSCLE RELAXATION (PMR)

PMR is one of the most popular relaxation exercises. It involves the systematic tensing and relaxing of specific muscle groups throughout the body.

PMR was invented by a physician, Edmund Jacobson, in the 1930s. Jacobson believed that the body tenses its muscles in response to anxiety and that it is impossible to be relaxed in body and anxious in mind at the same time. PMR is about letting go of emotional and physical tension and helps us to be more in tune with what our bodies are telling us.

The benefits of regular use of PMR include:

- Slower pulse.
- Reduced blood pressure.
- Slow, deep breathing.
- Reduced anxiety.
- No painful tension in the muscles.
- A sense of calm.

How to start each PMR session

- Remove restrictive clothing or spiky jewellery and ensure you are warm enough.
- Lie on the floor or a comfortable, supportive surface, although PMR can also be done sitting up. Try not to fall asleep – this does not help your relaxation skills!
- Practise on an empty stomach – the digestive process can interfere with relaxation.
- Start the exercise with 10 deep breaths, concentrating on your breathing.

The exercise

Start with one foot (it doesn't matter which). Breathe in, clench the toes tightly, hold for five seconds. Then breathe out, letting go of the tension. Relax for about 20 seconds then repeat with the other foot.

Move throughout the body, thinking about your breathing and feeling the tension disappear.

Legs – Straighten your legs and flex your feet (pointing the toes upwards and the heels towards the floor). If you're lying down, tense your thigh muscles by pulling the kneecaps up towards your hips.

Buttocks – Squeeze together and relax.

Stomach – Push out, making it as firm and round as possible. Relax. Then squeeze in tightly and relax.

Chest – Breathe in, hold for a few seconds then relax.

Hands – Clench your fists and relax.

Arms – Bend your elbows and tense your arms, feeling the tension in your upper arms.

Getting the most out of your PMR sessions
Practise for at least 20 minutes each day. Last thing at night is very helpful if you have problems sleeping.
Be careful when tensing any part of your body, and treat your neck, back and spine particularly gently.
Sit quietly for a few minutes afterwards. Your blood pressure can drop during relaxation and jumping up immediately afterwards could make you dizzy.
Visualize being in a calm and safe place to help you feel stronger in stressful situations.
Breathe in when tensing the muscles and breathe out when relaxing.

GETTING RID OF PHYSICAL TENSION

Try these other exercises to release tension in your body:

Shoulders

- Shrug your shoulders up towards your ears then relax.
- Pull your shoulder blades together and relax.

Back

- If you're lying on your back, leave your shoulders and buttocks supported and arch your back as you tense it, noticing where it curves most.

Neck

- Press your head back and bend it slowly from side to side (rolling the neck is not recommended!), noticing how the tension moves.
- Turn your head to one side as far as you can. Hold for five seconds, then relax, returning your head to the centre for ten seconds, feeling the difference in the muscles. Repeat, turning your head the other way.
- Move your head forward, tucking your chin in. Hold for five seconds and relax for ten seconds, feeling the difference. Return your head to its normal position.

Face

- Clench your teeth and relax.
- Push your bottom teeth in front of your top teeth.

- Frown and relax.
- Push your eyebrows up into your hair.

Has all the tension gone? If not, tense and relax again until you're sure that it's all disappeared.

Autogenic Therapy (AT)

AT was discovered in the early 20th century by Dr Schultz, a Swiss psychiatrist and neurologist. It's now very popular as a relaxation technique all over Europe and Japan.

Autogenic comes from the Greek words *'auto'*, meaning self-administered and *'gen'* meaning produce. It literally means a therapy you do yourself. The exercises, which are carried out in a state of 'passive concentration', are designed to switch off the body's stress-related 'fight and flight' system and encourage rest and relaxation. The attention is focused on sensations associated with relaxation (such as heaviness in the limbs or regularity of the heartbeat).

Studies have shown that regular use of AT helps reduce blood pressure, cholesterol levels and the risk of heart attack, as well as alleviating other stress-related conditions. Initially, AT requires specific instruction from a qualified practioner (see page 188), although it's available on the National Health Service in parts of the United Kingdom.

POSITIVE VISUALIZATION

Many people find that visualization (forming a mental picture of something pleasant) helps them to relax. Let's see if it works for you…

It's best to do your visualization in a quiet place free from interruptions! Imagine a place or an event that you remember as being peaceful, safe, happy and beautiful.

- Picture the place. Is it sunny? Are there waves lapping against the shore? Are you on a mountain?
- Think about the smells associated with that place or event… can you smell freshly-mown grass, the saltiness of the sea, a barbeque or someone's perfume?
- Next, think about the sounds….what can you hear? Waves, seagulls, music, laughter, children's voices – or is there complete silence?
- What can you taste? Crisp white wine – maybe your favourite chocolate?
- What can you feel? A warm breeze? Or cool water all around you as you swim in a deserted cove?
- Who is with you? Are you alone, with friends and family or a favourite pet?

This place can be your own special retreat from stress, so use it as often as you need to. You can also imagine stress flowing away from your body into the sea or up into the sky. As your body reacts to the scenes as if they were real, you should really relax.

Just pause...

Initially, you may feel uncomfortable about practising relaxation or positive visualization exercises. Or perhaps your busy mind won't allow you sufficient time and space to relax? That's by no means unusual. If that's the case, though, try pausing a few times during your day to encourage your mind to stop thinking about anything in particular – and simply slow down. Many opportunities occur naturally throughout the day that could enable you to do this, such as when you are:

- Cleaning your teeth.
- Waiting for the kettle to boil.
- Waiting for your toast to cook.
- Waiting at traffic lights.
- Waiting for the train/bus.
- Standing in a queue.
- Booting up your computer.

Try to slow down the pace at which you do everything, too. Eat and drink more slowly, walk more slowly, trying to take in more of your surroundings and savouring the moments. Why make your life a race to beat self-imposed and often unachievable targets?

Living a more relaxed life

Don't waste energy needlessly. Focus your attention on the four cornerstones of your life that need it (as discussed in Chapter 1).

Keep up the relaxation exercises. This is your defence against stress and pressure. Every day you will improve and be able to slip into a relaxed state anywhere, however busy and noisy your surroundings might be.

Regularly go back to our relaxation quiz on pages 39–41 to check how relaxed you are.

Allow yourself to recover from illness or physical and mental exertion so you are fresh and alert. If you're over-burdened in any area, shift your priorities or say no. If saying no is difficult, think about some assertiveness training.

Life shouldn't be a battleground, so try agreeing with people a bit more!

Always listen to what your body tells you. If you're under pressure, counteract it by whatever means works for you – relaxation or physical activity, or preferably both!

Are you making changes to help you relax? Answer the questions in the opposite table honestly...

	Yes	No
1) Do you understand why relaxation is important to your wellbeing?		
2) Do you set aside time each day for a relaxation or visualization exercise?		
3) Do you recognize physical tension?		
4) Do your muscles feel relaxed after exercise?		
5) After relaxation, do you feel:		
a) More in tune with your body?		
b) Calmer?		
c) You have a slower heartbeat?		
d) Your breathing is deeper and slower?		
e) Clearer headed?		
f) More optimistic?		
Score one for each 'yes' answer and each benefit in Q5), giving a total score of 10.		
Your total		

Your score

7–10 points – Well done! Keep up the good work.
4–7 points – You're feeling better, which is great. Carry on with the exercises.
3 points or less – Re-read the chapter, choose an exercise and do it each day for a week, and see how you feel then.

5-MINUTE FIXES: THE BODY

BODY AWARENESS, EXERCISE AND POSTURE

In this chapter you'll learn how to use exercise and correct posture to help release tension. By the end of the chapter you'll understand more about your body, what it's saying and why you must NEVER ignore its warning signals. If any of the recommended exercises cause pain, please stop doing them.

Did you know that your body responds to how you think, act and feel? This is called the 'mind-body connection'. Your body tells you when things are not right – usually when you're stressed, upset and anxious. And, as you've already seen, these feelings of 'not being right' manifest themselves as high blood pressure, insomnia, digestive upsets, fatigue and other symptoms.

Poor emotional health can weaken the body's immune system, making you susceptible to illness. Incorrect posture can make things worse, too, as you slump or contort your body into positions that cause tension and pain in the joints and muscles. Listening to your body is worthwhile, because doing so can encourage you to rest, helping to prevent illness, or enabling a quicker recovery.

Listening to your body

How well do you listen to your body's signals?Tick each answer that applies to you in this quiz:

1) When you're in the car, how do you sit?

a) Hunched over, gripping the steering wheel.
b) Leaning right back, almost horizontal.
c) Sitting up straight with head and back fully supported, hands relaxed on the steering wheel.

2) How often do you exercise?

a) Regularly – at least 3 times a week. You enjoy it so it fits in well with your routine.
b) About once a week because you're busy.
c) When you remember, which isn't that often.

3) How do you lie in bed?

a) On your front with your neck twisted.
b) On your back.
c) On your side.

4) How do you sit at the computer?

a) With the chair adjusted at a new workstation.
b) With the screen at eye level.
c) Interspersed with regular breaks.

5) How do you stand?

a) On the balls of your feet, stomach in.

b) On all parts of the foot with arms and hands hanging loosely.

c) Rigid with knees locked and chest out.

6) How do you release body tension

a) By going for a good workout at the gym.

b) By having another row with your partner.

c) You don't release it – ever!

7) How often do you do PMR each week?

a) You haven't had time to try it.

b) You've done it a couple of times this week.

c) You've done it each day.

8) Name three benefits of good posture.

a) Improved health.

b) You can run faster.

c) More confidence.

d) Better balance.

e) Reduced physical and mental tension.

f) Bigger muscles.

Score two points each for 1c), 2a), 3c), 4a, b or c) 5b), 6a), 7c), 8a, c, d, e)

Your total

Your score

20–26 points – Well done!You're already listening to your body and treating it well. Keep up the good work – but do read the rest of the chapter because hopefully you may learn something new and useful.

15–20 points – You're doing quite well already. Now read the rest of the chapter thoroughly and try out the tips in areas you scored less well in. Keep up the momentum, too, in areas you scored highly in.

10–15 points – It's not easy, but you've made a start. Read the chapter a couple of times and pick a different area to concentrate on each week. Even small changes can make a big difference to your overall health – and you will start to see the benefits quite quickly.

Below 10 points – You need to make some changes. Try reading this chapter several times and familiarizing yourself with the information. Then focus on a couple of areas you would like to change first – but don't make too many changes at once. If you are having particular difficulties with posture, for example, contact the Society of Teachers of the Alexander Technique, The British Chiropractic Association, or any other organization mentioned later in this chapter, for help. Their details start on page 186.

UNDERSTANDING THE MIND/BODY CONNECTION

There's a very strong connection between posture (how you move) and the state of your emotions. So:

- You smile or laugh when happy.
- You hang your head when depressed.
- You hunch your shoulders when scared.

You've probably noticed yourself that when you adopt postures indicative of a certain feeling, you do actually experience that feeling. Everyone feels happier when they smile, for example. So how does this work? Muscular contraction acts to hold the emotion/feeling within you and the movement and posture associated with that emotion or feeling can become a habit. Once this happens, you'll often find yourself in that emotional state. That can be good, or bad, depending on the posture, but the consequences are immense because this affects:

- The structure of your body.
- How people perceive and respond to you.
- Your overall attitude to life.
- Your emotional health (and relationships), because it can lead to suppressed emotions which are always bubbling under the surface needing to be let go.

BODY LANGUAGE

Body language, or non-verbal communication as it is also called, is a great example of the mind-body connection at work. How you act can reflect your emotions, causing you to send powerful messages to others, often without being aware of it. In essence, body language is to do with how people express themselves without saying anything, and it is made up of the following elements:

- Appearance (what you're wearing, how smart or scruffy, tall, short, muscular, fat or thin you are).
- Posture (which can convey your attitude (interest, respect, lack of interest or anger).
- How you walk (confident or shuffling), sit (slouching or upright), how you use your hands.
- Facial expressions and how you make eye contact.
- How you speak (tone of voice, pitch, accent, volume).

Did you know that what you actually say accounts for less than 10% of your communication? The other 90% is all about how you use your body. So being able to read body language is extremely important. Once you can interpret the behaviour of people around you, you'll have a much better understanding of how they think – and potentially remove a major source of stress in your relationships.

Reading body language

How well do you read body language? Find out with this quick quiz, ticking the answers that apply to you:

1) If the person you're talking to has their arms crossed and legs pointing away from you, do they feel:

a) Cold.

b) More relaxed.

c) Defensive.

2) If someone copies your actions, are they.....

a) ...trying to wind you up?

b) ... agreeing with you?

c) ...disagreeing with you?

3) What are the signs that someone is lying

a) Lack of eye contact.

b) Smiling.

c) Exaggerated hand movements.

d) Rubbing their nose.

4) When you meet someone for the first time, which do you most notice?

a) How they sound.

b) How they look.

c) What they say.

5) In the Mediterranean which one of the following indicates companionship?

a) Eye contact.

b) Using hands to gesticulate.

c) Laughing a lot.

6) Which one of the following could help you succeed in a job interview?

a) Nodding.

b) Raising your voice.

c) Steepling your hands.

Your total

Your answers: Score two points each for answering:

1c) If people have their arms (and legs closed) this usually means they're feeling negative. Uncrossed arms and legs indicates you're relaxed and open.

2b) If you're getting on well with someone you often mirror each other's postures unconsciously. If you lean forward, they will do the same, and you'll both probably pick up your drinks at the same time, too!

3a, d and e) give these answers two points each. They're all indications that lies are being told. Other give-aways include biting fingernails and a guarded posture (such as folded arms).

4b A recent study indicates that we notice appearance (55%) over what people say (7%), or how they sound (38%).

5b In Mediterranean Europe, eye contact is seen as friendly, but in the UK it can indicate aggression or attraction if prolonged. So, when you're abroad be careful about how you act, as you can unwittingly cause offence by *not* making eye contact, just as you could in the UK by making too much.

6a Nodding your head, smiling or a firm handshake conveys a favourable impression to potential employers. Unfortunately, steepling hands implies you're over-confident and a know-it-all.

Your score

10–16 points – You can interpret others' body language. Now look at what messages you're conveying!

6–10 points – Practise reading others' body language by watching how people act with each other at parties or in restaurants.

5 points or less – Don't worry if you're finding this difficult. Re-read the chapter a few times and watch out for examples of the behaviours we've discussed, not forgetting about your own non-verbal communication!

EXERCISE TO BEAT PHYSICAL TENSION

For stressed people regular exercise is one of the best ways of getting rid of pent-up tension and stale emotions.

The benefits of exercise

- Stronger heart, lower blood pressure (and levels of blood cholesterol) and improved circulation.
- Better quality sleep.
- Stronger immunity to illnesses like colds and flu (by lowering levels of cortisol which switches off the immune system).
- Reduced anxiety and a greater sense of calm.
- Reduced depression and a feeling of wellbeing via 'feel-good' chemicals.
- A wider social circle.
- A distraction from problems.
- Increased longevity.
- Loss of excess weight and promotion of toned muscles, which help improve confidence.
- Improvement in memory and concentration.
- It's fun!

Why does exercise help?

Exercise helps drive out stress hormones such as adrenaline and cortisol, and encourages the production of 'feel good' chemicals like endorphins (responsible for the 'runner's high'). Exercising increases our oxygen intake and white blood cells – which help fight illness – increase temporarily after exercise.

Which exercise is best?

That depends entirely on you! It's best to choose an exercise you enjoy (because you're more likely to do it regularly) and one that will provide physical release.

Do bear in mind that exercising itself should not cause you stress. It can – if it becomes too competitive or you stop enjoying it. If that happens, you could perhaps either take a more laid-back approach or try something else.

There are so many different activities to choose from nowadays. Some, like tai chi and yoga are gentle, relaxing and meditative, although yoga also helps strengthen and tone. Swimming is an excellent choice if you suffer from back and joint pain, because you're fully supported by the water. With its emphasis on good breathing and correct spinal and pelvic alignment, pilates can help you become more in tune with your body.

Weight training, kickboxing and all the martial arts are especially good choices if you have plenty of pent-up frustration to release!

Exercising safely

f it's been a while since you exercised regularly, ease your body in gently with some walking or swimming. You can then work up to more vigorous exercise if you wish. People who do too much exercise too soon risk injuring themselves – the joints and lower back are especially vulnerable. They're also more likely to give up when progress is slow. The following should help you get the best out of your chosen activity:

How to make the most of your exercise

Check with your GP first that it's safe for you to exercise.

Exercise regularly for 20 minutes at least three times a week for best results.

Choose something you enjoy, which fits easily into your life. You're more likely to keep it up.

If winning is important to you, avoid competitive sports like tennis, squash or football – they could increase your stress levels!

Always warm up before exercise, and stretch afterwards, to acclimatize muscles and joints.

Strong abdominal muscles can help prevent a bad back, so think about doing some stomach exercises.

Build more exercise into your daily routine.

Always listen to your body and NEVER ignore pain!

CORRECTING POSTURAL ALIGNMENT

According to the British Chiropractic Association, the ideal posture allows *'for a plumb line to hang straight through your ear, shoulder, hip, knee and ankle. Try and stand relaxed, but gently contracting your abdominal muscles. When sitting the same is true, the gravity line should pass thorough the ear, shoulder and hip.'*

Good posture is extremely important. Most people don't give a second thought to sitting, standing or

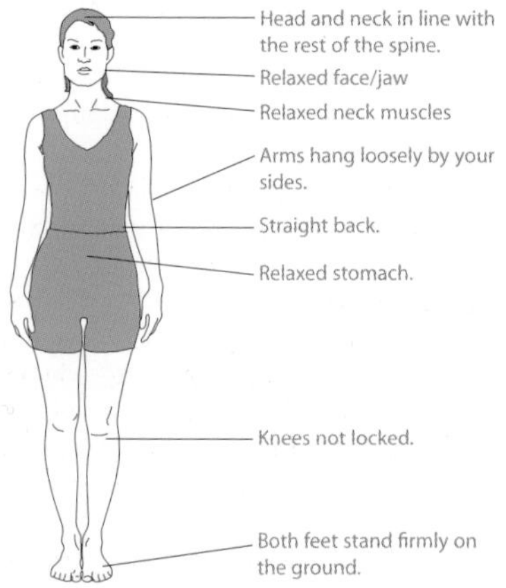

Correct postural alignment.

walking. But in actual fact how they do all these simple, everyday things has a huge impact on their physical and mental well-being.

Good posture means standing tall, walking tall, and sitting tall. It makes you look and feel good, and your body work more efficiently. It puts the least amount of strain on the ligaments and joints in the spine, pelvis, and legs.

Some benefits of correct posture are:

- Improved health, appearance and coordination.
- Increased strength and stamina.
- Your clothes fit better.
- You have more confidence and better body balance.
- Reduced possibility of injury.
- Improved physical and mental development.

It's the job of the skeletal muscles (which are attached via tendons to bones) to cause and control movement and help maintain posture. As you learned in Chapter 2, muscles work in pairs and in opposite directions. For a movement to occur, one group must contract while the other must stretch.

It is important that opposing muscle groups are balanced in strength, especially if they are postural muscles. If not, an imbalance can occur where one side is stronger, and you'll tend to hold yourself and move in a way that uses the strength of stronger muscles and ignores those that are weaker. This results in poor posture, because the skeleton is pulled out of shape by the muscles.

So, you can be literally locked into positions that cause pain and stress. When you slump in front of your television set, computer or behind the steering wheel of your car, you're pulling down the muscles in the neck, throat, jaw, chest, abdomen and upper thighs.

There can be many reasons for poor posture:

- Injury.
- Poor sleep support/position.
- Spinal and pelvic misalignment.
- Emotional problems.
- Being overweight.
- Eye problems.
- Poor nutrition.
- Foot problems (a foot injury may cause you to stand and walk differently, potentially straining your leg muscles and affecting your back).
- Weak muscles.
- Negative mental and physical attitudes.
- Recurrent occupational stress/position.

Effects of poor posture

Condition	Reason why	Effect
Muscles more prone to injury.	Muscles/tendons weak with lack of use and vulnerable if used suddenly/vigorously.	Pain.
Poor circulation in the muscles.	Lack of movement and sustained muscle tension.	Lethargy/ tiredness.
Poor waste removal	Lack of blood flow so muscles don't get enough oxygen and glucose for energy release. Waste builds up, with cells less able to carry out tissue repair.	Pain/slow recovery from injury.
Shallow, inefficient breathing.	A posture restricting the expansion/contraction of the ribcage. Inefficient use of lungs.	Lethargy/ tiredness.
Pain in the nerves.	Muscle tension irritates nerves travelling through muscles.	Pain.
Overuse of stronger muscles.	They're often contracted and become tight. They are difficult to relax/stretch, remaining tense.	Pain and general tiredness.
Under-use of weaker muscles.	They rarely contract so become flaccid and prone to injury/poor circulation	Muscle sags, fat builds up.
Emotional repression	Negative emotions are locked into particular postures.	Depression/ emotional tension.

THE ALEXANDER TECHNIQUE

According to the principles of the Alexander Technique, released, lengthened muscles work more easily and effectively than tight ones.

A century ago, Frederick Alexander, an actor, discovered that if he freed or released his neck muscles, his head, followed by his body, could release in an upwards direction without undue effort. This guiding principle can be applied to any movement. By teaching you to direct and organize your body properly, the Alexander Technique can help you regain a healthy posture (although you'll need to consult a qualified teacher) and also to:

- Be more co-ordinated.
- Move easily.
- Be alert and focused.
- Be calmer and less tense.
- Be energetic without too much effort or tension.
- Be more self-aware.
- Waste less energy.
- Avoid discomfort and strain, preventing bodily wear and tear.

Releasing postural tension

Tension can quickly build up in our bodies as a result of sustained poor posture. The following tips should help minimize the risk of this happening, although some people experience a greater impact by following this advice than others do:

Adopt postures that need little muscular effort to maintain. These use the bones to take the body's weight, so that all the muscles have to do is to maintain balance rather than holding the body in shape against the force of gravity. This means:

- Balancing the head so its weight travels down the neck rather than having the head slightly tilted (forwards/backwards/sideways) or having the chin jutting forwards.
- Allowing the shoulders/arms and hands to relax and dangle when not actively being used.

Move and/or adjust your posture regularly when still. Sitting or standing still for long periods causes circulation to grow sluggish and inefficient (leading to lack of nutrients and oxygen in the cells, poor waste removal, poor repair of wear-and-tear, faster ageing and tiredness.) And if muscles have to work to maintain the posture, they become tired, tense and painful.

TIP: Shoes can help maintain good posture. For walking and overall regular use, swap shoes with thin, high heels for soft-soled shoes, which are supportive and have a good grip.

CAREFUL CARRYING

Avoid shoulder bags as these pull down the muscles on one side of the body. Instead, opt for a bag (like a rucksack) that puts equal weight onto both shoulders. Adjust the straps so that it is close to the back and the weight is evenly distributed.

Check your bag/briefcase each day, taking out items you won't need, otherwise your neck, shoulders and back will carry unnecessary weight!

Try this Alexander Technique exercise to release postural tension:

1) Pile several books on a firm surface, like the floor, and lie down, resting your head on them. They must be the right height for your neck – and this will vary from person to person. If they are too low, your head will fall back and down. If they're too high, your larynx will be restricted.
2) Allow your spine to be supported by the floor, placing your arms beside your body and bending your knees so your feet are flat on the floor.
3) Stay there for at least 10 minutes, thinking about how your body is feeling.
4) Roll your body to the side and get up gently.

STANDING COMFORTABLY

Proper body posture while standing (as well as walking, sitting and lifting) is essential, and can help prevent and control lower back pain as well as other distortions in the body. Try the following advice from the Society of Teachers of Alexander Technique:

1) Stand on all parts of the foot. Keeping your heels in contact with the ground is important, because sensory nerve endings in the heels send your brain vital messages about balance. The point of your heel should line up with the three outer toes, pointing forward.

As a general rule of thumb, stick to the three-points standing rule, which is basically a triangle, standing on the:

- Heel.
- Outer edge of the foot behind the little toe.
- Ball of the foot behind the big toe.

2) Your knees should be relaxed, and your arms and hands hanging loose by your side. Your shoulders know where they are supposed to be, so they will position themselves naturally.
3) Walk tall! The weight of the head is supported by the neck, and you should be thinking 'forwards and upwards', with no muscular effort at all.

The following exercise will help you to stand more comfortably – and with a good posture:

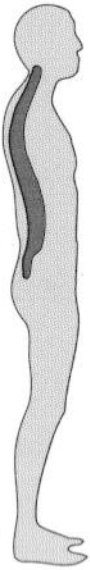

Stand straight,without leaning forwards, backwards or sideways.

Think about being forward and upwards.

Shoulders, arms and hands are relaxed.

Pelvis relaxed and straight.

Knees relaxed.

Both feet on the ground.

Standing correctly.

Some dos and don'ts for standing comfortably:

Don't try to squeeze in your stomach, as by doing this you're trying to correct something that's wrong anyway and you'll just create more tension.

Don't pull your shoulders back.Doing this will narrow your back, creating tension in the shoulders and in the upper chest.

Don't teeter on the balls of your feet – you will lose balance!

Don't lock your knees or your pelvis will tilt backwards.

Do move around periodically to boost your circulation.

If you have to stand for a long period, a footstool will help relax your ankles and knees, providing you change the foot you're standing on regularly.

WALKING COMFORTABLY

Any advice people get on improving their fitness usually includes adding a walk to their exercise regime. Have you ever thought about how you walk? Probably not, because it's something you're supposed to do instinctively. Most people spend a lot of time walking, but too often they do it wrongly – resulting in pain and tension. So what is the right way to walk?

The foundation is good posture. Think about a line extending from the top of your head and let it direct you. Your head should be supported forwards and upwards, but not leaning forward. Leading with your head will put you out of balance. Your legs will have to catch up and your shoulders will come up to protect your head in case you fall – leading to further tension. You should look forward, at least three metres in front of you, not down to the ground. If you need to look down, move your eyes, not your head. Tilting your head forward strains the neck and shoulders.

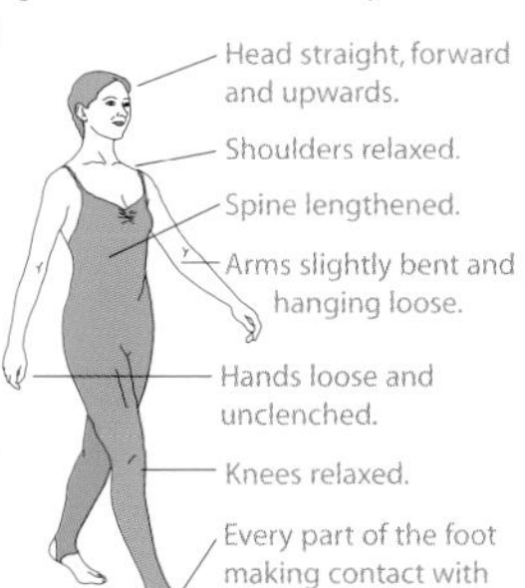

Walking correctly.

Shoulders, arms and hands

When you are walking, relax your shoulders and let your arms swing freely with each step.They should be preferably slightly bent rather than being totally straight. Your hands should be relaxed and loosely closed, not clenched, as this will cause tension. Your spine should be lengthened by standing tall and straight, but relaxed.

Legs and feet

Don't think about how far you're getting with each step.Think about getting a good stretch on the calf and the stride as being an extension of the hip and joint.The knee automatically bends and your foot will swing forward, taking with it your body. Visualize thinking up through the front of the spine, the real centre of your body.

The best way to walk

- Head straight, forward and upwards.
- Shoulders relaxed.
- Spine lengthened.
- Arms slightly bent and hanging loose.
- Hands loose and unclenched.
- Knees relaxed.
- Every part of the foot making contact with the ground.

SIT UP STRAIGHT

Many of us spend a lot of our working day sitting – at desks, in meetings, in cars, on the train. When we get home, we relax – often by sitting in front of the television!

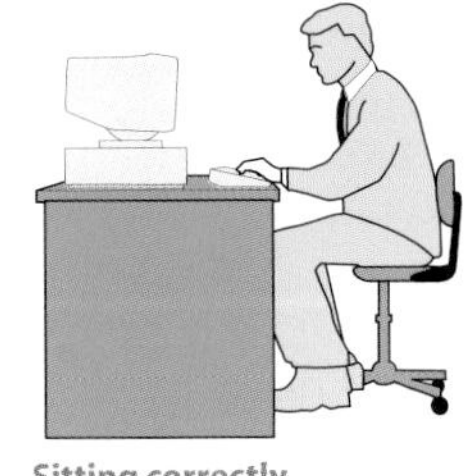

Sitting correctly.

Do you ever think about how you're sitting? Try this exercise:

1) Sit in a chair. Notice if you're slouching or sitting upright.
2) Stand up. Was it an effort?

Now try again – the Alexander Way.

3) Sit upright, your head is supported upwards and, at the same time, allow it a little 'nod' forwards.
4) Think about freeing your neck, imagining a line travelling through the top of your head.
5) Stand up, by leaning forward, tilting that imaginary line so it directs your body up and forwards.

Did that feel any better?

Sit up straight – at your computer

Do you spend most of your working day in front of a PC? If so, it's vital that you sit comfortably and that your spine is fully supported.

The following tips should help you to work comfortably and avoid injury:

- Always adjust your chair when moving to a new workstation.
- Ensure that your chair supports your back and that your hips are slightly higher than your knees. Your shoulder blades should be touching the back of the chair.
- Make sure that your computer terminal is at eye level so that you don't have to strain your neck looking down.
- Always take regular breaks, usually after a half hour, even if this is just for a couple of minutes. Look away from the screen, into the distance, to relieve eye tension.
- Don't collapse your wrist when using the keyboard.This can cause tension in the arms, repetitive strain injury or carpal tunnel syndrome.
- Your feet should be placed flat on the floor or on a footrest. Always make sure you have enough legroom under your desk.

Sitting up straight – in the car

For most people, posture is not uppermost in their minds when driving. But you should consider it – your back is under twice as much pressure when you're sitting incorrectly as when you're standing! A correct driving position reduces stress on the spine and is, of course, much safer. Here are some tips for comfortable driving using the Alexander Technique:

- Sit right back in the seat so you're fully supported.
- Adjust your seat so that the height and incline are right for you. If the seat is too low, there's a gap between your thigh and the seat, resulting in an over-extended ankle and calf strain.
- ALWAYS position the head-rest correctly – this could prevent whiplash if you have an accident.
- Gripping the steering wheel causes arm and neck tension. Instead, rest the heel of your hand on the wheel, using the little finger and ring finger to steer.
- If you change gear, turn your hand in the direction of the gear change rather than forcing it. Don't grip the gear stick with the thumb, do it gently with the heel of the hand and outside fingers.

TIP: If your car seat is uncomfortable or does not offer enough adjustments to enable you to get comfortable, invest in seat accessories from a motoring superstore.

Sit up straight – in front of the TV

A great deal of the nation's time is spent in front of the television – more often than not slouching, unfortunately.

The ideal sitting position is to let your chair or sofa take your weight. If possible, you need to keep as much of your body in contact with the chair so that your whole body is supported. You can place extra cushions in the small of your back or behind your neck if you feel you're not getting enough support.

Don't crane your neck towards the television set. This will cause head, neck and shoulder tension, and will place further stress on your back. It could also cause eye-strain, especially if you need glasses and are not wearing them, or are sitting too close to the TV set. On page 85 we offer some useful tips on how to release (and avoid) eye strain.

TIP: The above advice holds good for watching anything for a long time – whether you are at the cinema, the theatre, a concert, attending a work presentation or watching live sport. Be aware of your seated posture as you watch – it will mean you are more comfortable in the long term.

LYING DOWN COMFORTABLY

Just as there are many ways of sitting up, standing or walking (not all of them correct!), so there are different ways to lie down.

In bed

On average, we spend seven hours asleep each night, so the correct sleeping position is important.

- Adopt a sleeping position which creates less stress in the back – lying on your side rather than on your front with your neck twisted.
- When you wake up, do a few gentle stretches, such as drawing your knees to your chest and slowly rolling from side to side.
- Invest in a good quality mattress and pillow. Most experts believe that a mattress should mould itself to the body. Brands like Tempur offer mattresses and pillows in materials that sense body weight and temperature and adapt accordingly. Many chiropractors and osteopaths believe these can ease and prevent back and neck problems, reduce tossing and turning and promote a good night's sleep. But, the most important thing about a mattress is that it is supportive. Many people find Tempur mattresses too soft and too hot – so there's no such thing as a cure-all mattress!

Resting your spine

It's important to rest your spine regularly if you suffer with back problems. The best way to do this safely and comfortably is to lie on a firm surface (such as a carpeted floor) with the knees slightly apart and bent, and feet firmly on the ground. Not only does this prevent pressure on the lower back, but it also helps lengthen the spine.

Lie with your head on a pile of books (see page 72) or with a small pillow, cushion or rolled-up towel beneath your neck. Place your arms gently by your sides, palms open.

If you're lying with your legs on the ground, you can put a cushion or pillow under your lower back and knees to reduce strain on the back or the pelvic area.

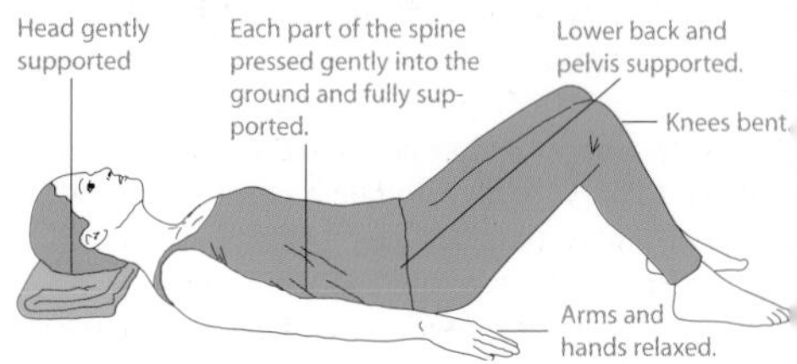

Resting your spine.

RELEASING HAND TENSION

Hands are vital tools, and are used for many essential tasks at home and at work – typing, writing, gardening, housework, driving, playing an instrument, to name just a few.

Hands get tense like any other part of the body and people – like typists, musicians or factory workers – who repeatedly perform certain movements, are especially vulnerable to repetitive strain injury (RSI). Symptoms include weakness in the wrists, tingling fingers, aching muscles, pain and even an inability to use the hand.

Regular release of tension is therefore very important. Try the following Alexander Technique exercise:

1) The muscles of the fist are situated below the crook of the elbow, on the inside of the arm. These muscles contract when you grip something.
2) Think about releasing those muscles and lengthening through the carpal tunnel (inside the wrist) to the tips of the fingers.
3) Long tendons (cords of fibrous tissue connecting muscles with bones) run from the muscles in the forearm to the fingers. Think of the wrist as a busy junction box which needs to be kept wide and free of tension.

RELEASING EYE TENSION

Do you spend hours reading or at your computer? Are your eyes screwed up and strained? At work most things you'll look at are close up and so you don't generally look into the distance. The following exercise will help you release built-up tension in the eyes:

- Think about widening, releasing and softening the muscles around the eyes.
- Be aware of your peripheral vision.
- Think about your surroundings, place yourself mentally.
- Look away from the computer screen every 20 minutes, into the distance, out of the window if possible.
- Don't screw up your eyes. What you see isn't at the surface of your eye – the visual centre is actually in the brain, at the back of the head.

More tension relievers

If you need a bit of extra help in getting rid of muscle tension, have a go at these simple exercises:

1) Sit in a chair with your feet squarely on the ground and your arms relaxed and resting gently on your legs.

2) Turn your head from let to right and down, very slowly and gently, feeling the stretch in your neck. When your right ear is as close to your right shoulder as it will go, return your head gently to the central position.

3) Now do the same exercise, this time stretching your neck from right to left. How did that feel? Would you like to try something different?

4) Still sitting down, pull both shoulders up and rotate them five times from the front to the back. Repeat the same exercise five times, circling your shoulders from the back to the front.

TIP: Squeeze a soft juggling ball several times a day to keep your hands supple and reduce the risk of developing stiff joints and tendons. It's also a great stressbuster!

FEEL BETTER NOW?

Have you implemented any of the tips suggested in this chapter? If you have, do you feel better? If you have not, is there any particular reason why? Try re-reading the chapter once more to see if any of the tips could apply to you. It may also be a useful exercise to re-do the questionnaire on pages 55–6 and see if your scores have improved at all.

5-MINUTE FIXES: BREATHING

This chapter looks at how human beings breathe, how they should breathe to maintain optimum health and why correct breathing is so important. It also has several exercises to help you improve your breathing, including one for dealing with panic attacks. Let's look at what you already know about breathing, ticking the answers that apply to you.

1) How do you feel about your breathing?

a) I don't give it much thought.

b) I focus on it when I remember.

c) I try to be aware of my breathing as it can tell me when something's not right.

2) How do you sit sit at your computer?

a) Hunched over, breathing rapidly.

b) Upright, breathing from your abdomen.

c) Yawning a lot?

3) Where's your diaphragm?

a) In your chest.

b) In your stomach.

c) Between your chest and stomach.

4) Do you do breathing exercises to control the rhythm of your breathing?

a) Yes, I do one every day.

b) Yes, I do them when I have time.

c) No, I'm much too busy.

5) Name three benefits of breathing correctly:

a) Stimulating mental alertness.

b) Being calming and relaxing.

c) Building up muscles.

d) Improving coordination.

e) Maintaining the correct balance between the gases in the blood.

f) Giving your nose a work-out.

6) How do you breathe when you walk?

a) I haven't really noticed.

b) I breathe as usual, but it's not very deep.

c) I take in big lungfuls and exhale as much as I can.

7) Name three symptoms of a panic attack

a) Slowing heartbeat.

b) Sweating.

c) Fainting.

d) Pins and needles.

e) Trembling.

f) Ear ache.

8) How many times do you breathe each minute?

a) 20 times.

b) 6 times.

c) 10 times.

Scoring your answers – give yourself two points each for: 1 (c); 2 (b); 3 (c); 4 (a); 5 (a, b, e); 6 (c); 7 (b, c, e); 8 (c)

Your total

Your score

20–24 points – Good for you! You already know a lot about your own breathing mechanism, why it's important and are generally breathing correctly.

15–19 points – You're doing pretty well. Now try to practise a breathing exercise at least once a day.

10–14 points – You're getting some things right. It can take time to change years of improper breathing habits. Try to implement the tips in this chapter but take it slowly – lots of small changes can build up into big ones, so remember that if you feel you're not making progress!

9 points or under – Re-read the chapter, focusing on one breathing exercise and do it once a day. If you keep this up, you will make solid progress. Why not try a yoga class? The British Wheel of Yoga (see page 186) can provide details of a class local to you.

HOW DO WE BREATHE?

Breathing is vitally important to our survival. It's possible to live without food for a few weeks and water for a few days, but we would die without air.

Most people breathe in (inhale) and out (exhale) without understanding what they're doing. Breathing is the movement of air into and out of the air passages. It's a complicated mechanism, involving the use of the lungs, thorax, diaphragm muscles and the intercostal muscles (situated between the ribs).

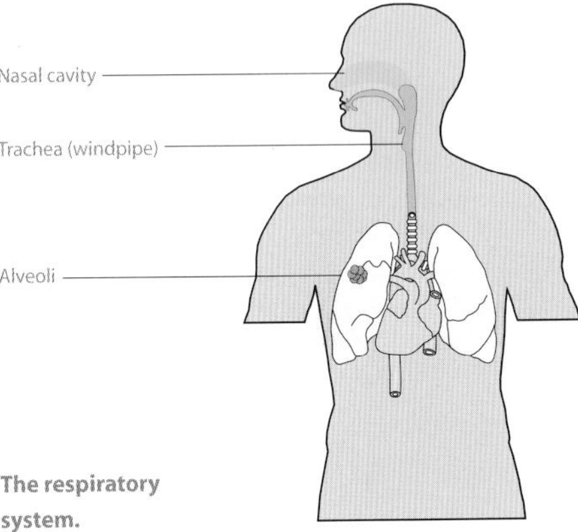

The respiratory system.

The act of inhaling sets off a chain reaction that lowers the diaphragm and raises the ribs. This increases the volume of the thorax (containing the heart and lungs, protected by the ribcage) and draws in oxygen.

When you inhale, air enters through your nose and mouth where it is warmed to body temperature and becomes moist. The increase in water content is important in helping to prevent the lung tissue from drying out.

The air then passes through the trachea to the lungs, which inflate. It is in the tiny alveoli of the lungs that oxygen finally meets the bloodstream. Each alveoli has a network of blood capillaries through which oxygen is transported (to the heart), and where oxygen and carbon dioxide are exchanged.

Breathing correctly

Various chemical reactions occur in which oxygen is used to break down glucose into carbon dioxide and water, causing a release of energy. Called internal respiration, this process occurs in all body cells. The by-product – carbon dioxide – is carried back to the lungs where it is then exhaled.

The role of the diaphragm

The diaphragm – a thin layer of muscle separating the thorax from the abdomen – is vital to the breathing

DID YOU KNOW THAT?

- A normal breath (inhalation plus exhalation) takes four seconds.
- Adults breathe 12–18 times per minute, about 22,000 times a day.
- We inhale and exhale 14,000 litres of air per day.
- The surface area of the alveoli on a pair of lungs could almost stretch over an entire tennis court!

mechanism. It contracts each time you inhale, moving downwards. This increases space in the chest cavity, allowing air to flow deep into the lungs.

When you exhale, your diaphragm moves upwards, reducing chest space and pushing air out.

Generally most people don't breathe deeply enough to engage their diaphragms. Instead, they breathe using just their chest, neck and shoulder muscles, which inflates the upper area of the lungs only, rather than filling their full capacity. Because they take in just small amounts of air, they have to breathe more. That's tiring – and bad for the posture, dragging on the head, neck and shoulders.

Your respiratory system (the breathing mechanism) is closely linked with your cardiovascular system (relating to the heart and blood vessels) and both work together to provide your body cells with oxygen for energy release.

Taking in enough oxygen – and expelling the right amount of carbon dioxide – is vital in sustaining good health. If this doesn't happen, stress can occur because the body has to work harder to maintain its chemical balance, and breathing may quicken, potentially triggering off the fight or flight response. As I explain later in the chapter, many of us breathe too much ('over-breathing'), which can lead to panic attacks and some forms of asthma.

The benefits of deep diaphragmatic breathing include:

- Reducing tension and stress.
- Helping control panic attacks.
- Being relaxing and calming.
- Stimulating mental alertness.
- Helping in efficient waste removal.
- Helping stimulate your body to produce endorphins ('feel-good' chemicals), linked with our perception of pain and possibly involved with controlling emotions and mood.
- Exercising your lungs by using more of your lung capacity.

HOW SHOULD WE BREATHE?

Proper breathing when you're resting involves using the abdomen and diaphragm, rather than the chest. It means relaxing the neck, shoulder and chest muscles , taking air into the bottom of the lungs. When you exhale, you draw in your abdomen slightly, which encourages an increase in abdominal tone. This type of breathing is deep, slow and effortless, and helps maintain a good posture. The body automatically adjusts the amount of air you take in and the rate at which you breathe. But it's still possible to over-breathe using the diaphragm.

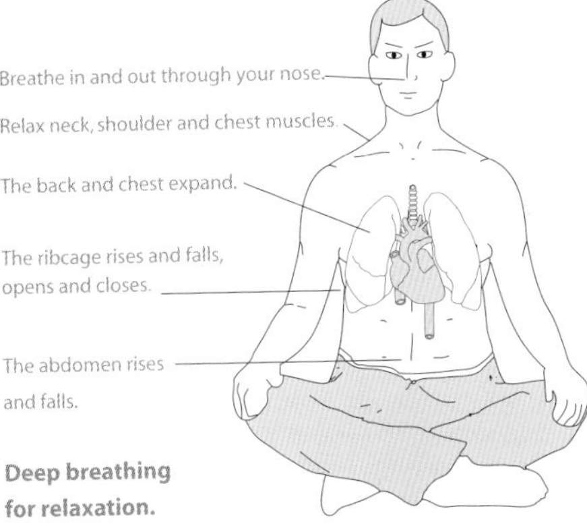
Breathe in and out through your nose.
Relax neck, shoulder and chest muscles.
The back and chest expand.
The ribcage rises and falls, opens and closes.
The abdomen rises and falls.

Deep breathing for relaxation.

CONTROLLING THE RHYTHM OF YOUR BREATHING

Focusing on your breath and its rhythm is very relaxing. Other benefits of controlling the rhythm of your breathing, by counting for example, include:

- It stills the mind and, in turn, your breathing will also settle.
- As your mind and body relax, your breathing slows down, as does your heartbeat, and your nervous system will calm.
- This exercise can be helpful before practising deep relaxation or meditation.
- It could also help you get a good night's sleep!

Mentally counting the breath

Try the following exercise:

1) Observe your breath for a few moments, allowing your breathing to stabilize.
2) Each time you breathe in and out (and without changing the rhythm of your breathing) count how long each inhalation and exhalation takes. It doesn't matter how long each one is – you're merely observing, not judging or altering.
3) Notice if your in/out breath changes with each breath. After a while, though, your breathing rhythm should settle down naturally, so that each

successive inhalation takes the same length of time, and so does each successive exhalation.

4) Don't worry about counting any pauses that occur after inhaling/exhaling. Just enjoy feeling the peace and stillness between counting.

Alternate nostril breathing

This is one of the most popular yoga breathing exercises. It relaxes and calms the mind, relieves tiredness and is said to balance the body's vital energy.

1) Sit comfortably. Place the thumb of your right hand by your right nostril and its fourth and little fingers by your left nostril (it's probably easier to tuck the index and middle fingers into your palm).
2) Close your right nostril using your thumb and breathe in through your left nostril to a count of seven. If seven is too long, inhale/exhale for as long as is comfortable.
3) Close your left nostril with your fourth finger. Release the thumb and breathe out through your right nostril to a count of seven.
4) One you've finished breathing out, inhale through the same nostril to a count of seven, so…
5) Close your right nostril with your thumb, release your fourth finger and exhale from your left nostril to a count of seven.
6) Continue doing this for 10 minutes and repeat twice daily, if possible.

DEEP BREATHING EXERCISES

By allowing your breath to flow naturally, you become aware of the rhythm of your own breathing. It's soothing and calming, and you relax mentally and physically. Not only do you 'concentrate' in a relaxed way (as in meditation), but you become more attuned to your body. Have a go at the following exercise:

Inhalation/exhalation

1) Lie or sit down comfortably. Don't slouch!
2) Close your eyes (to help you concentrate on your breathing).
3) Put one hand on your ribs and the other on your stomach.
4) Breathe in through your nose – for as long as you can – and allow the air as far down into your lungs as possible.
5) Exhale through your nose, slowly and evenly – for as long as it took you to inhale – or longer if you can manage it. If the out-breath is longer than the inhalation, this stimulates the part of the nervous system responsible for relaxation.
6) Notice how many breaths (inhaling and exhaling together count as one breath) you do each minute and repeat.
7) Observe the feelings and sensations associated

with your breathing:

(a) Can you feel cold air going in and warm air coming out?

(b) Does your abdomen move outwards or your ribcage rise when you inhale?

(c) Does your abdomen draw in on the out-breath?

(d) Is your breathing smooth and regular?

(e) What do you feel in the pause between exhalation and inhalation?

(f) Can you hear air flowing out when you breathe?

Getting the most out of your breathing exercises

Avoid breathing exercises for two hours after a heavy meal.

Discomfort interferes with breathing – so ensure you are as comfortable as possible.

Wait until 30 minutes after strenuous physical activity when your breathing has returned to normal.

Don't do the exercises when ill, hungry, depressed or tired.

If you feel dizzy or light-headed, stop, and try again next day. These are warning signs of hyperventilation (see pages 98–101).

Do the exercises regularly. The more often and the longer you practise, the greater and quicker the benefits!

BREATHING TO REDUCE ANXIETY

As we saw in Chapter 1, how calm or agitated people feel is controlled by the autonomic nervous system – and this process is also closely linked to breathing. Being angry, upset or frightened triggers various physical and mental changes. For example, your heart will beat faster and your blood pressure rises. Your breathing also changes, becoming quicker than usual and losing its natural rhythm. The action of breathing faster increases your agitation, so you breathe even faster – and so begins a vicious circle.

Such over-breathing is known as hyperventilation. Over-ventilating the lungs (by breathing too fast or too deeply), causes an excess of carbon dioxide to be flushed out of the bloodstream.

The level of carbon dioxide in the blood matters. It influences the acid/alkaline balance of the blood and its presence is needed during the transfer of oxygen from the red blood cells to the body.

When sensors in the blood vessels detect low levels of carbon dioxide, the body automatically narrows the air passages to the lungs and tightens the muscles involved in breathing – to reduce the number of breaths that you take.

The body's attempt to force shallow breathing can make you feel like you can't breathe, and the increased tension in your breathing muscles just heightens your general feeling of stress.

By this time the vicious circle is firmly established. Stress has caused your breathing to quicken, leading to physiological changes which push your stress levels up further – and the fight or flight response rears its ugly head again! Of course, there's usually nothing to fight or run away from. But if you don't release the tension via physical activity, those stress hormones keep flooding your body and cause even more stress.

Increasing the speed of your breathing suddenly can result in frightening symptoms like palpitations, dizziness and chest pains (caused, not by a heart attack as some people believe, but by a spasm of the muscles between the ribs).

When you're relaxed, your breathing is usually gentle, slow and rhythmic. It is possible, therefore, to use your breathing to become more aware of your mental and emotional state – and to change that state. You can use your breathing to slow and calm yourself. So, when you're anxious, you should simply breathe more slowly (but not more deeply, as that can lead to hyperventilation).

HYPERVENTILATION AND PANIC ATTACKS

On the previous two pages we discussed how stress can quicken your breathing, which in turn increases stress, beginning a vicious circle. When all those stress hormones are in full flow, people can experience extreme anxiety and feelings of panic. They are, in fact, having a panic attack. Most attacks are accompanied by hyperventilation – and having too much oxygen can bring about unhelpful bodily changes.

Symptoms of a panic attack:

- Excessive sweating, especially in the hands and underarms.
- Feeling sick.
- Increased anxiety.
- Rapid heartbeat.
- Dizziness.
- Light-headedness.
- Hyperventilation and shortness of breath.
- Chest pains.
- Dry mouth.
- Trembling.
- Fatigue and weakness.

Sometimes the person having the panic attack faints. Clearly this is very distressing, both for them and for anyone witnessing the attack. However, fainting can be nature's quick-fix solution. It enables the body to stop breathing for a very short while, stabilizing the gas levels in the blood and eventually restoring the body to equilibrium.

Breathing during a panic attack

Have you ever had a panic attack where you hyperventilated because you felt you couldn't breathe? You were experiencing an abnormally low level of carbon dioxide that your body couldn't cope with – caused by over-breathing. The following techniques are tried and trusted ways of beating hyperventilation:

Overcoming hyperventilation

Holding your breath. Hold your breath for as long as you comfortably can. Repeating this several times will quickly stabilize the balance of oxygen and carbon dioxide in your body, steady your breathing and calm you.

Breathing into and out of a paper bag. This may look odd, but it's really effective! Inhaling the carbon dioxide you've just exhaled will stabilize the oxygen/carbon dioxide content of your blood.

Taking some strenuous exercise! A brisk walk while breathing through your nose (and exhaling deeply through your mouth) is very calming. Regular exercise also reduces tension.

BETTER BREATHING WHEN MOVING

Be aware of your breathing while you are moving. While you are walking, breathe in deeply, using your diaphragm and abdomen, so you get as much air as possible into your lungs. Try to exhale for as long as you can, to expel all that stale air. Then begin to synchronize your breathing with the pace of your walking. Your breathing will probably change depending on the nature of your exercise. Any activity that involves moving quickly, such as jogging, football, squash, dancing and many others, will increase your body's need for energy, so you will have to breathe in more oxygen.

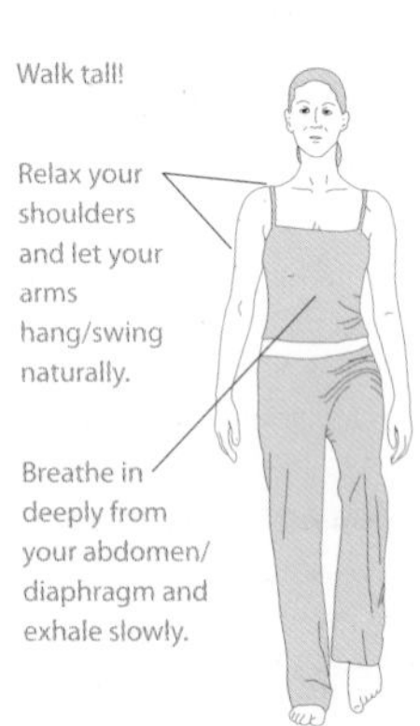
Walk tall!
Relax your shoulders and let your arms hang/swing naturally.
Breathe in deeply from your abdomen/ diaphragm and exhale slowly.

Breathing on the move.

Your breathing will be deeper and faster, and can be affected for up to 30 minutes after exercising. Remember to warm up before exercise, and cool down and stretch afterwards, taking some deep breaths to calm your mind and body.

BREATHING AT WORK

If you're hunched over your desk, peering at your computer screen, the chances are that you're not breathing properly. Do you sigh or yawn during the day? That could be a sign that your breathing is too shallow and you need more oxygen. Shallow breathing, combined with caffeine, lunch on the go and anxiety about deadlines or that meeting with the boss can be a pretty devastating combination. As well as cutting down on caffeine and eating more healthily (see Chapter 6), a breathing exercise in your lunch hour will set you up nicely for the afternoon ahead. It relieves stress, and may even make you more productive!

1) Breathe in deeply, dropping your chin towards your chest.
2) Gently raise your head to its usual position, while breathing out.
3) Repeat as many times as you like.
4) Stretch your arms over your head, taking a deep breath.
5) Hold your breath, stretch for a few more seconds, then slowly release the stretch and your breath.
6) Repeat the same breathing pattern while you alternately stretch your arms out in front, then behind you.

BREATHING FOR DEEP RELAXATION

As you learned in Chapter 2, the regular practice of deep relaxation can help protect you from the ill effects of stress, and may also reduce the symptoms of stress-related diseases. It can also increase your overall ability to cope. How are you doing with the Progressive Muscle Relaxation exercise? If you weren't sure how to breathe during this exercise, read on…

How to breathe while doing PMR

You can lie or sit while practising PMR. When you're comfortable, let your breathing settle down into a slow rhythm. Don't actively try to breathe deeply – just be aware of how your stomach rises and falls. As a general rule of thumb, breathe in while you're tensing your muscles and relax them when you breathe out. Ensure that every part of your body is relaxed before finishing the exercise. If there's still a tense area, repeat, remembering to breathe correctly. When you're finally relaxed, keep your breathing slow and regular.

Shavasana and body awareness

When you're relaxing, why not try a classic yoga pose like Shavasana? Shavasana releases tension, strengthens your back, arms and legs, stretches the abdomen muscles, slows down the heart and breathing rate and can reduce overall stress and fatigue.

Before you start, check the following:

- Are your toes relaxed, your legs loose but straight?
- Move your fingers, relax your arms and shoulders, roll your head from side to side.
- Keep your head straight.
- Lie still for a minute, trying to detach your mind.

Then, inhale deeply and begin to bring awareness to each part of the body, not consciously tensing or relaxing it. Begin with your left toe and ending with the top of your head. Try to direct your breath to each part as well. Once you're fully relaxed, you can use other deep relaxation techniques such as visualization or a breath awareness exercise. Remain in the pose for about 15–30 minutes in total. If you feel yourself drifting off, breathe more rapidly.

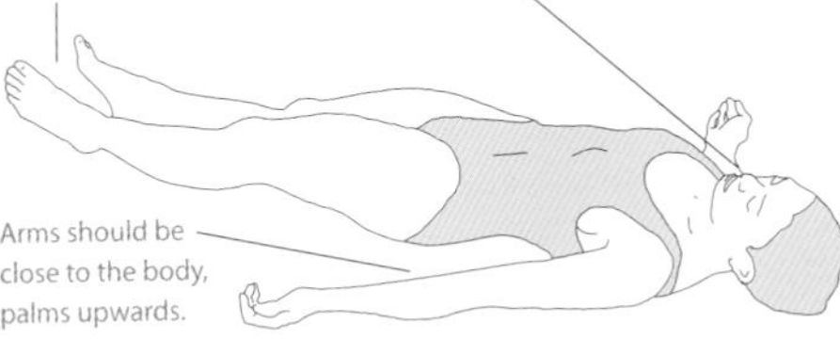
Feet should roll out naturally with legs about 18 inches apart.
Breathe deeply and evenly through nostrils.
Arms should be close to the body, palms upwards.

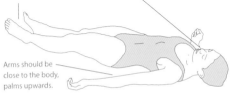

Proper breathing position for deep relaxation.

MAKING THE MOST OF BREATHING EXERCISES

The following tips may help you make the most of your breathing exercises:

1) Try to breathe through your nose (unless you are suffering from some condition which prevents you from doing so – a cold, for example.) Unlike the mouth, the nose warms up the air in preparation for entering the lungs. It also filters out dust and germs, and that's important because the tissue of the lungs is delicate and easily irritated

2) It's useful to have a routine both before and after breathing exercises to settle your attention and awareness on your breath. Try the following:

Before your breathing exercise:

- Go to the toilet, even if there's just the slightest need.
- Loosen any tight clothing.
- Always make yourself completely comfortable before you begin, adopting a relaxed posture with an elongated spine.
- Have a blanket to hand in case you get cold.
- Use a relaxation technique and stretching to remove tension.

After your breathing exercise

- Be quiet and still for a while, enjoying how you feel.
- Draw your awareness to where you are, what's happening and what you'll be doing next.
- Give yourself a positive message like 'I'm going to open my eyes and get up feeling refreshed'.
- If you're too relaxed to move, increase the depth of your breathing until you feel like moving.

Tip: Try sighing/exhaling the breath through the mouth two or three times to release tension. If you're really tense, breathe out noisily and sharply – preferably in private!

Asthma

This chapter has not discussed breathing with asthma. If you are asthmatic, you are probably already managing your condition under medical supervision. You may also be using the Butekyo breathing techniques which can be helpful. If you think you may be asthmatic, do not attempt the exercises covered in this chapter and go to see your GP.

Tip: To check if you're using your diaghram (as opposed to your upper chest area), feel below your breastbone at the top of your abdomen. Cough slightly and you should feel the diaphragm push out, moving as you breathe.

5-MINUTE FIXES: STRETCHING AND MASSAGE

Regularly stretching and massaging the muscles can work wonders in helping you to relax. It dispels pent-up tension in problem areas (such as the neck and shoulders), and can also improve the overall flexibility of our muscles. That's important because it can help avoid injury.

The most popular exercise/stretching systems (such as Yoga and Pilates, for example,) recognize the importance of how the mind and body can work in harmony together. They combine exercise and stretching with deep breathing to still the mind and give the body a good work-out.

How to stretch safely

- Warm up via gentle walking or marching on the spot before stretching. This increases blood flow and makes the muscles more supple.
- After exercise, walk around for several minutes to reduce your heart rate before stretching (otherwise blood can pool in the muscles, leading to possible cramp and dizziness).
- Hold the stretch until you feel the muscle loosen, then hold for a further 10 seconds.
- You should feel a little discomfort while stretching,

but always stop at the first sign of severe pain!

- Never bounce while stretching.
- Always breathe regularly throughout the stretch.

ANKLE CIRCLING

1) Stand up straight.
2) Lift one foot off the ground and circle it, first one way, then the other.
3) If you're overbalancing, hold onto something.
4) Now do the same with the other foot.

CALF STRETCH

1) Stand with one leg about 30cm in front of the other. Both legs should be straight but don't lock the knees. Both feet should face forward.
2) Lean forward, keeping the body straight.
3) Keep the back heel on the floor (you can bend the front leg slightly) and feel the stretch in the calf muscles at the back of your leg.
4) Hold for 10 seconds then swap legs.

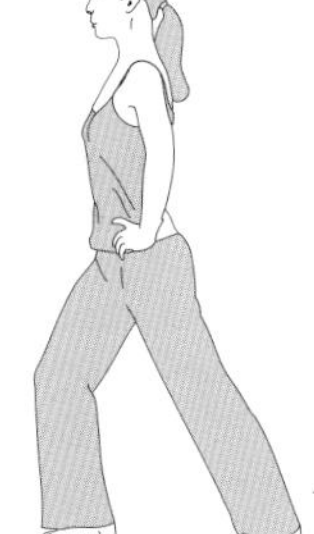

Calf stretch.

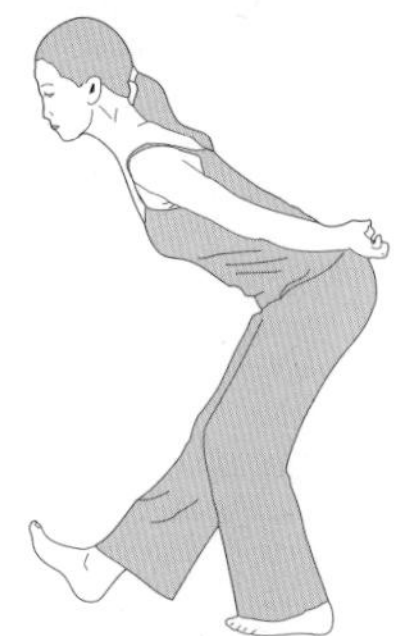

Hamstring stretch.

HAMSTRING STRETCH

1) Standing up straight, step forward with one leg.
2) Bend the knee of your back leg, keeping the front leg straight.
3) Keep the weight on the back leg, but lean forward, feeling the stretch at the back of your front thigh (hamstring). Always keep your back straight. You can rest your hands on your hips to help you balance.
4) Tilt your bottom upwards and hold for up to 10 seconds then swap legs.

CHEST STRETCH

1) Stand up straight.
2) Clasp your hands behind your back and slowly lift your arms upwards.

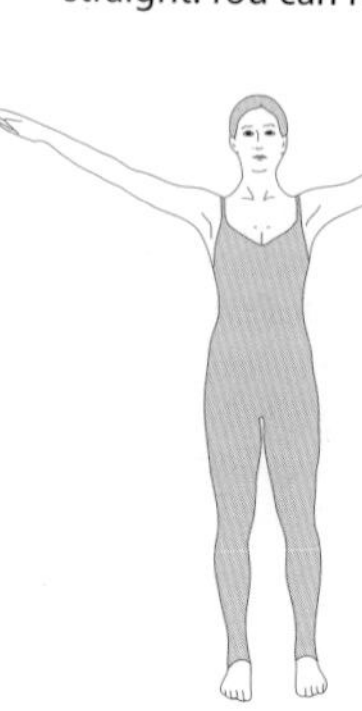

Chest stretch.

3) Squeeze your shoulder blades together and hold for up to 10 seconds, feeling the stretch in your chest and pectoral muscles.
4) If you can't clasp your hands, just reach behind you and lift as far as is comfortable.

INNER THIGH STRETCH

1) Sit up straight on the floor.
2) Open your legs as wide as is comfortable. Breathe in.
3) Breathing out, lean forward from the hips keeping the back straight. Do not be tempted to hunch over.
4) You should feel a gentle stretch in the inner thighs. Settle into the stretch, holding for 10 seconds, breathing regularly then exhale and return to your original position.
5) Repeat twice more.

LEG EXTENSION

1) Kneel down with your hands below your shoulders, breathing normally.
2) Inhale, lower your head and raise your left knee, curling your back towards the sky.
3) Lifting your head, exhale, straighten your left leg and push it out behind you, as high as possible. Your spine will automatically lengthen, keep it straight, thinking of it as a tabletop.
4) Hold for ten seconds, then relax and repeat with the other leg.

SHOULDERS AND NECK RELEASE

Tight neck and shoulder muscles can cause real misery, as anyone who's ever suffered from stiffness and aching in those areas (and the resulting throbbing headaches) knows! If you're a sufferer (and/or if you sit at a computer for long periods) performing the following exercises regularly could reap dividends.

ARM CIRCLES

1) Stand up straight.
2) Keeping your shoulders and arms loose, make large circles with your arms.
3) Do five going back and then bring forward five times.

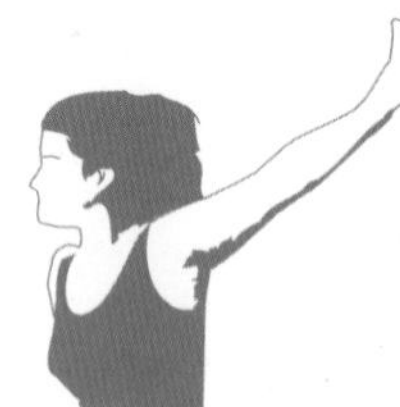

Arm circles.

ELBOWS BACK!

1) Stand or sit up straight, looking forward.
2) Breathe normally, putting both hands on your lower back

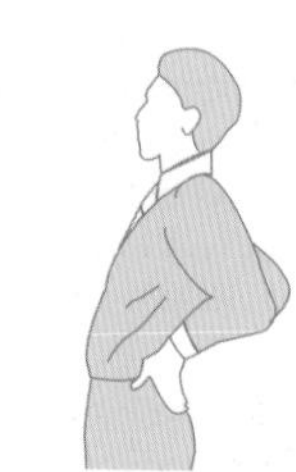

Elbows back.

with your elbows out to the sides.

3) Breathing out, pull the elbows back, trying to get them to touch.
4) Hold for 10 seconds.
5) Relax and repeat three times.

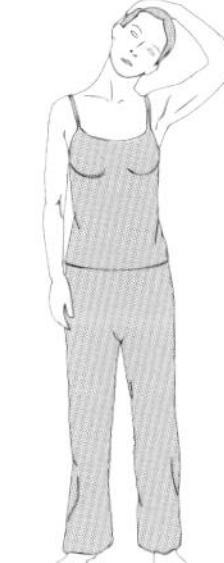

Neck and shoulder stretch.

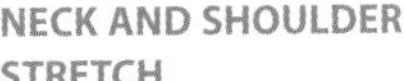

NECK AND SHOULDER STRETCH

1) Stand in a good posture.
2) Tilt your head to the left as far as you can, and push the right shoulder down as far as you can.
3) Put your left hand on the right side of your head – gently – and feel the stretch for 10 seconds.

SHOULDER ROLLS

1) Stand up straight.
2) Roll your shoulders backwards five times.This movement involves only the muscles of your shoulders **not** your neck.
3) Then roll your shoulders forwards five times.

TIP: The neck is very delicate so perform any neck exercises slowly and smoothly. Never, never jerk the neck.

STRETCHING TO RELEASE TENSION IN YOUR SPINE

The following are great exercises for letting go of tension in your spine and the muscles in your back.

EASY UPWARD STRETCH

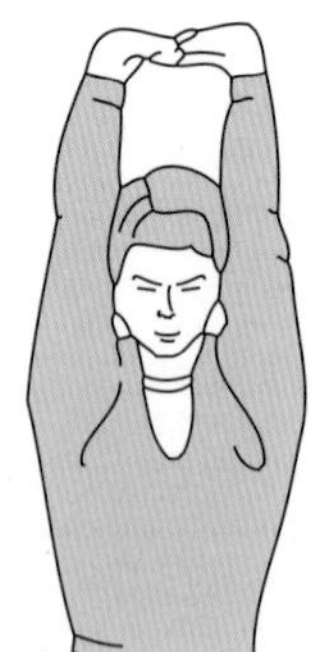

Easy upward stretch.

1) Stand up straight with both feet flat on the floor. Extend both hands straight above your head, palms touching.
2) Inhale, slowly pushing your hands upward, then backward, keeping your back straight.
3) Hold for 10 seconds, breathe out and relax for a few seconds before you repeat (five times).

Avoid this stretch if you suffer from back pain.

SPINAL RELEASE

This exercise isn't about touching your toes.

1) Stand up straight with your back against a wall and your feet shoulder-width apart, and inhale.

2) Bring your chin to your chest.
3) Exhaling slowly, gently curl the spine downwards, peeling each vertebrae away from the wall (but keeping your buttocks in contact with the wall).
4) Your knees should be gently bent and allow your hands to dangle loosely towards the floor.
5) When you've gone as far as is comfortable, breathe in and gradually straighten up, with your neck and head coming up last.
6) Repeat four times.

SIDE STRETCH

1) Stand straight with your feet shoulder-width apart, knees slightly bent and tummy tucked in.
2) Reach your right arm up and over your head to the left side, letting your left arm reach down your left leg to your knee.
3) Stretch down as far as you can and hold for five seconds. But be careful – if you feel pain, ease off.
4) Repeat with your other arm.

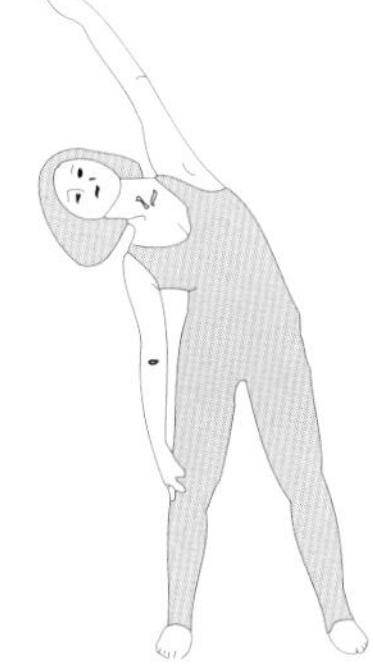

Side stretch.

SPINAL TWIST (FOR LOWER BACK FLEXIBILITY)

Avoid this if your lower back is weak or injured.

1) Sit up straight on a chair, feet flat on the floor and your hands gently resting on your thighs.
2) Pull in your stomach muscles and breathe regularly.
3) Gently and slowly turn your head to the left, to look over your left shoulder, letting your spine follow.
4) Breathe out as you do this and place your right hand on your left leg.
5) Slowly move back to your original position, ending up facing towards the front.
6) Repeat on the other side, turning your head to the right. Do this exercise five times on both sides.

CAT STRETCH (1)

1) Kneel down on all fours, pointing your fingers forward and your toes behind.

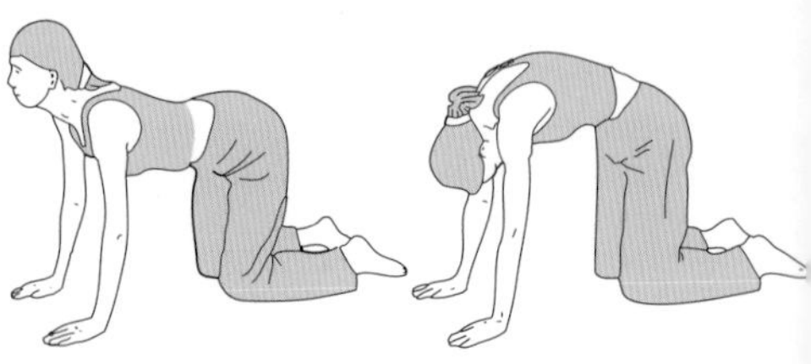

Cat stretch (1).

2) Ensure your back is straight and flat, like a table-top.
3) Drop your head downwards (but don't touch the floor), pushing your shoulder blades upward and outward so as you lift (round) your upper back.
4) Hold for 20 seconds, not forgetting to tuck your stomach in and breathe regularly throughout the exercise.

CAT STRETCH (2)

1) Kneel down on all fours, pointing your fingers forward and your toes behind.
2) Ensure your back is straight and flat.
3) Move your arms forward until your forehead touches the floor.
4) Hold for 20 seconds, breathing regularly, feeling the stretch in your shoulders and upper back. Release.

Care: Don't curve your spine – keep your back straight at all times!

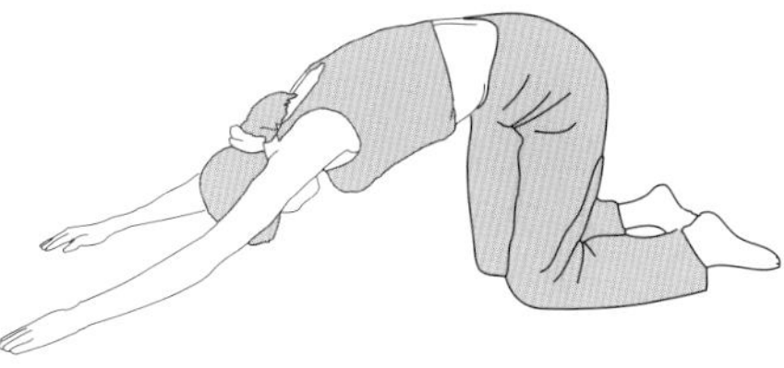

Cat stretch (2).

LYING TRUNK TWISTS

1) Lie flat on your back, with both hands straight out and inhale. Your legs should be either bent or straight and both resting on one side.
2) Exhale, sliding both legs up towards the arm, aiming to keep the knees together, while allowing

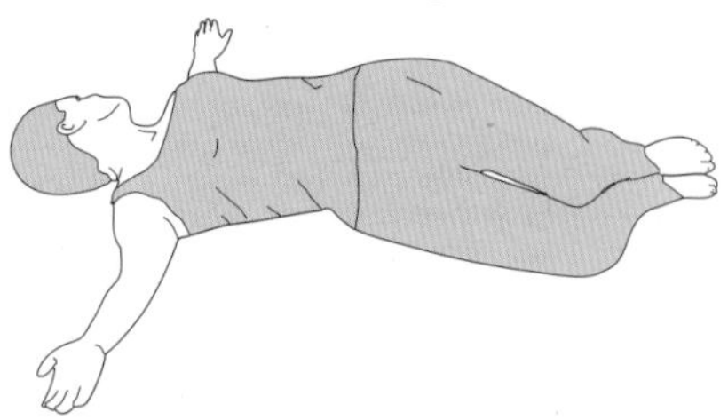

Lying trunk twists.

your lower body to twist round. (You can do this with your legs bent or straight.)

3) Remain in this position for 10 seconds, exhale and release. Repeat on this side twice more and then do the exercise on the other side.

TIP: Strong abdominal muscles will help protect your back from the stresses and strains of daily life, so try to firm your stomach muscles as much as you can.

STRETCHING TO EASE LOWER BACK PAIN

Pain in the lower back can be miserable. Curling the back can help ease pressure and relieve pain in that area.

FOETAL POSITION

1) Lie on your back, gently pressing your spine into the floor.
2) Keep your head on the floor and breathe normally.
3) Slowly pull both legs into your chest, and wrap your arms around the back of your knees.
4) Breathe out and pull down on your legs while gradually lifting your buttocks off the floor.
5) You can stretch your neck, once in this position, by slowly tilting your chin to your chest and holding for 10 seconds.
6) Gently return to your original position. Relax for a few seconds and repeat twice more.

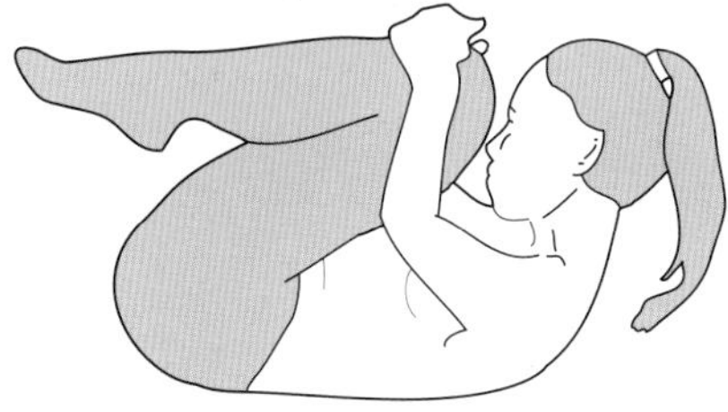

Foetal position.

FACIAL MUSCLE EXERCISES

Did you know that there as many as 44 muscles in your face? These can become as tight and sore as any others in your body. Exercising your facial muscles is one of the best ways to release tension. Just 5–10 minutes' exercise each day can promote a healthier-looking complexion, rejuvenate elasticity and natural collagen and smooth/lessen fine and deeper lines.

MOUTH WRINKLE PREVENTER

1) Open your mouth and make a large 'o'.
2) Hold your lips tightly over your teeth.
3) Then widen out to make 'eee' and 'oooo' sounds.
4) Repeat each one five times.

TONGUE PRESS (TO PREVENT/REDUCE A DOUBLE CHIN)

1) Keeping your mouth closed, press your tongue against the roof of your mouth, breathing normally.
2) At the same time, gently stroke your neck backwards and forwards, using your thumbs.
3) Hold for 20 seconds and relax. Repeat.

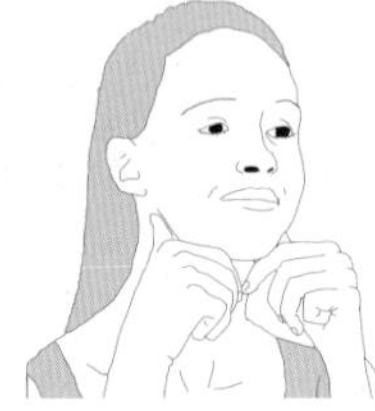

Tongue press.

MASSAGE

Massage is the act of kneading or rubbing the soft tissues of the body to improve circulation and aid suppleness and relaxation. It can be relaxing to both give and receive a massage.

Benefits of massage

- Improves circulation and reduces muscle tension.
- Helps to eliminate waste products via stimulation of the circulatory systems (cardiovascular and lymphatic), so oxygen and other nutrients reach the cells and tissues.
- Helps release endorphins, the body's own painkillers.
- Reduces anxiety and stress.
- Increases energy and vitality.
- Improves digestion.

SOME HINTS FOR GIVING/RECEIVING A MASSAGE

If you're having a massage, lie on a firm but padded surface.

The masseur (se) should wear flat shoes and remove rings.

If you're massaging, keep your back straight and use the weight of your body to give power to the massage.

Don't massage people who are ill, have back pain, skin infections or certain other conditions.

Massage firmly to invigorate, use slow steady strokes to relax.

FACIAL MASSAGE

Giving the face a workout can leave the person looking and feeling younger, as improved circulation brings back a healthy glow to their skin. It can also soothe away tension and pain in those 44 muscles! Ask the person massaging you to follow the contours of your face with their fingers (remembering to remove glasses or contact lenses before they start).

1) Your friend should make small circular movements at the temples with their thumbs, then widen to cover the whole forehead. Stroke the forehead from the nose to the hairline.
2) Starting at the temples,they should massage over the bridge of the nose, stroking out across the eyebrows, coming back under the eyes to the nose.
3) Make gentle circular movements around the mouth with the middle fingers of both hands, then stroke up each side of the face, one hand at a time.
4) Stroke under the jaw up to the ears. They should pause briefly with their hands over your ears, then bring their hands back under your chin.

TIP: Get into a routine of doing the exercises while watching the TV or doing household chores.

HEAD, NECK AND SHOULDER MASSAGE

This area needs particular attention because the shoulders and neck are often tense – not surprising since they have to support the 6kg (14lb) weight of the head! Your friend may have to work firmly on particular areas to get out the knots (small lumps caused by bunched muscle fibres or a build-up of waste) – and you may feel temporarily stiff and sore after the massage.

All that work will reap dividends because you will probably tingle in the massaged areas (these can also look quite red). Don't worry – those are good signs, meaning that the blood is beginning to flow back into the muscles.

1) They start by moulding their hands to your body and stroke from the top of your shoulders up to the top of your neck, and back down,

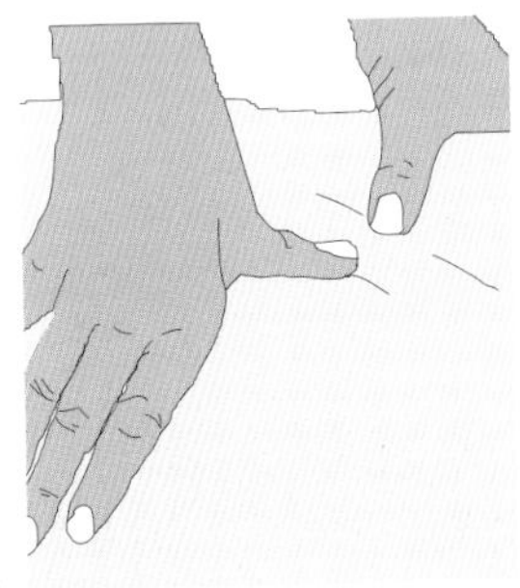

Step 1.

doing this several times.

2) Gently knead the neck muscles and the tops of both shoulders to get rid of all that tension.

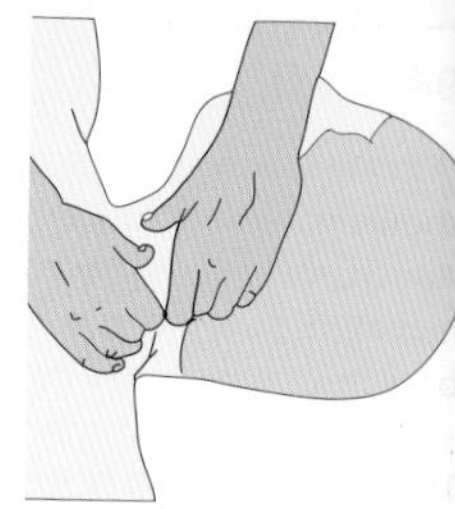

Step 2.

3) Gently sweep around the upper chest and continue the sweep up around the back of the neck.

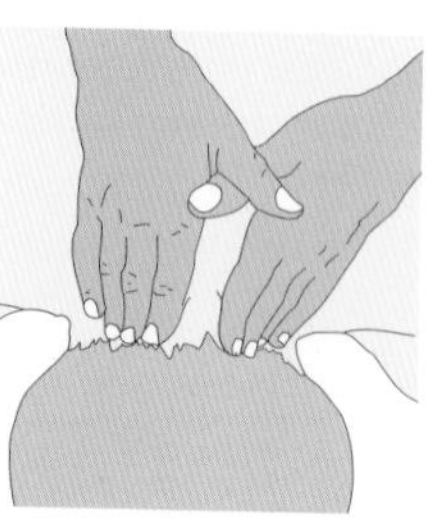

Step 3.

4) They should try working in circles, with their thumb on the side of your neck and their index, middle and third fingers on the other. Making small circular movements, press the muscles gently.

TIP: When massaging the neck and shoulders, the movements should be smooth, gentle and slow, otherwise you could end up with more tension in your muscles.

BACK MASSAGE

Massage can greatly relieve tension in the back and shoulders, often caused by carrying heavy bags or slouching in front of the computer or television. The human back contains many nerves – and a thorough back massage can soothe or invigorate them.

There are lots of different ways of massaging the back but the following are a few your friend can try:

1) Start at the lower back. They should mould their hands to the contours of your back, their thumbs on either side of your spine. Sweep up the back, working up towards the head and gliding back down, pressing firmly.

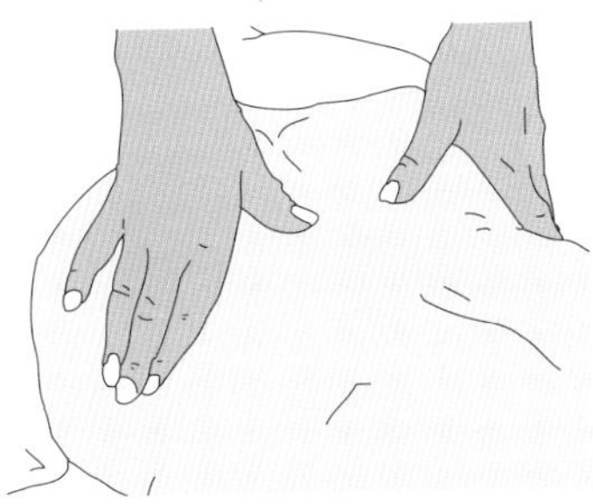

Back massage, step 1.

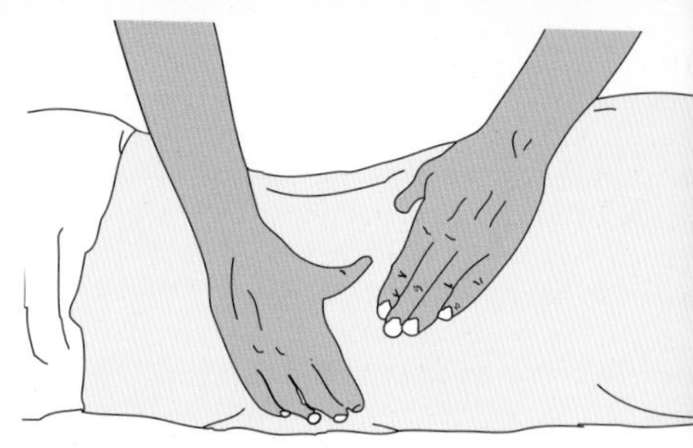

Back massage, step 2.

2) Grasp handfuls of flesh at the side and squeeze. Gently and rhythmically knead the flesh, starting at the hips, working up each side of the body, taking care not to dig or tickle.
3) Put both hands on the right hand side of the back, slightly apart and slide one hand down the side in a curved movement while the lower hand goes up towards the spine. Continue across the whole of the back.
4) Let's apply some pressure to relax the spine. Starting at the lower back, your friends should place both thumbs on either side of the spine, leaning to apply pressure. Press, release and then move up the spine until you reach the neck. They shouldn't press too hard – the spine is delicate.

) Let's try some circle thumb stroking. Put both thumbs on either side of the spine and stroke round in a small circle, moving up the body.

) For side stroking, stroke up the sides of the body pulling towards the spine. One hand should follow the other in a slow, steady rhythm.

) Fan stroking is a variation on the original stroking movement we did in step 1 (illustrated on page 125). Your friend should put their hands on your lower back and stroke up towards the neck, pressing on the muscles on each side of the spine. They can then move each hand out in a fan shape over the top of the back and glide lightly down the sides of the body.

) They can start and finish a massage using these two moves, (8) and (9) – sliding their hands down each side of the spine, fanning them at the bottom of the ribcage towards each side of the body.

) Move their hands up the sides of the body bringing them in and under the shoulder blades and back, out over the top of the shoulders, bringing them to rest at the back of your neck.

TIP: Your friend should try kneading slowly for a relaxing massage, increasing the tempo of their movements for a more invigorating massage.

FOOT MASSAGE

The foot is an incredibly complex mechanism, designed to take the weight of the whole body. It contains about 25 per cent of the body's bones and numerous muscles, tendons and ligaments.

A foot massage can be very relaxing. The sole of the foot contains thousands of nerve endings and the whole body can be stimulated by massaging these.

1) Get your friend to stroke the foot firmly in upward strokes from the toes to the ankles. This is very warming and relaxing.

2) Support the foot with both hands and, with their thumbs, stroke in between each of the grooved

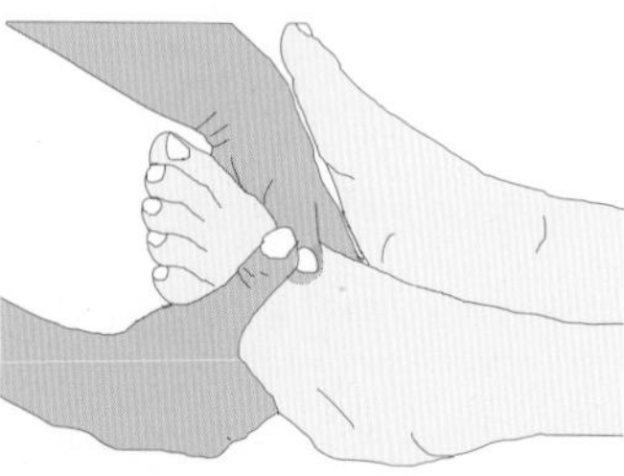

Foot massage, step 1.

areas between the tendons (running from the ankles to the toes), doing at least three strokes.

3) Moulding their hands around the foot which is sandwiched between their hands, they should sweep up and over the sole gently, from the base of the foot, including the instep, arches and heel.

4) While supporting the heel of the foot with one hand, they should use the other to massage each toe. Squeeze gently, rolling each toe in both directions, then pull it gently towards them.

5) Stroke up the foot gently, fanning out towards each side and smoothly gliding back towards the toes. This is very calming and relaxing for the recipient. Now repeat steps 1–5 on the other foot.

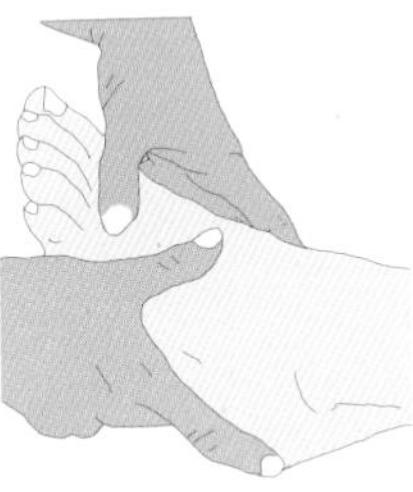

Foot massage, step 2.

SELF MASSAGE

If you don't have anyone to give you a massage, you can do several basic versions yourself quite easily. These can increase your circulation, release tension, boost your energy levels and give you a feeling of vitality. So, let's get started!

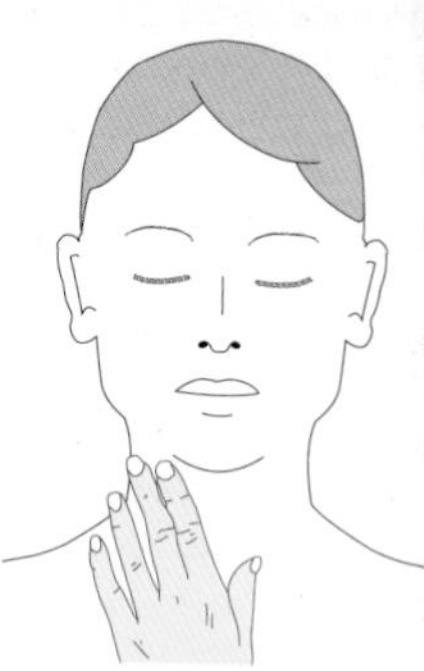

Self massage, Step 1.

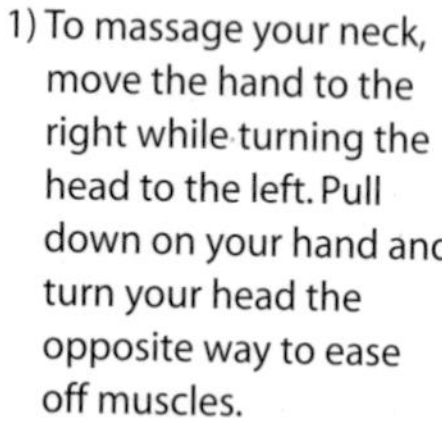

1) To massage your neck, move the hand to the right while turning the head to the left. Pull down on your hand and turn your head the opposite way to ease off muscles.

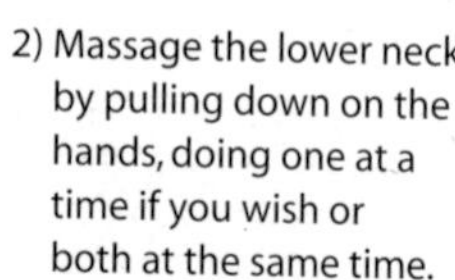

2) Massage the lower neck by pulling down on the hands, doing one at a time if you wish or both at the same time.

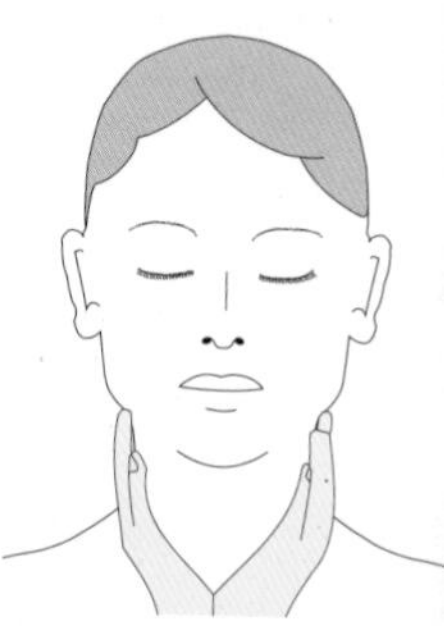

Self massage, Step 2.

3) Sweep up the chin from the base of the neck. Strokes should be firm to stimulate circulation and this can help keep your neck looking younger.

4) Use overlapping strokes to massage the face gently.

5) Make circular movements on your arm with your thumb. Follow this by squeezing the flesh all the way up your arm and back again. Then stroke firmly up the arm from wrist to shoulder and back again.

6) Bend forward, place your hands into the small of your back and then lean back into them.

7) Massage your knees in circular movements with the tips of your fingers. Sweep up behind the backs of the knees towards the thighs. Knead the thighs, squeezing and releasing the flesh, and then pummel them with your fists to increase circulation.

8) Stroke your feet all over. Then work on each toe individually, pulling it gently to give it a good stretch, then releasing. This is wonderfully relaxing.

TIP: You can buy self-massage DVDs which will show you all the moves you need in the privacy of your own home.

Massaging your hands

Our hands work hard each day, especially if we have to type or perform any other repetitive manual task on a regular basis. Tension can quickly build up in your hands, so give them a pampering massage every now and then.

1) Place your hand palm up in your other hand, supporting it at the back with your four fingers.

2) Using small circular movements, press all over the palm of your hand with the free thumb, moving up to massage the wrist and back down again.

3) Repeat on the other hand.

4) With your thumb, stroke between the tendons on the back of your hand, from the knuckles, all the way up to the wrists.

5) Repeat on the other hand.

6) Hold the fingertip between the index finger and thumb of the other hand, and pull gently to stretch it.

7) Repeat for each finger on that hand.

8) Swap hands.

FEEL BETTER NOW?

By now, you should feel able to perform a few simple stretches to ease tension out of your body. You may, of course, choose to join a yoga or pilates class, with the added bonus of meeting like-minded people. As we already know, socializing is one of the best ways to relieve stress.

The most important thing is to do the exercises regularly. Make them part of your routine and they will become another chink in your armour against stress. The added bonus, of course, is that they will help increase your overall levels of fitness, which will also make you feel better about yourself.

With regard to massage, there are many qualified masseurs/masseuses. The General Council for Massage Therapy can help you find a reputable therapist in your area (see details on page 189).

Tip: If you're having a back massage, remember that lying on your front with your head to one side can strain your neck. So always put a small cushion or rolled-up towel under your forehead.

5-MINUTE FIXES: EATING

WHY WE SHOULD EAT HEALTHILY

Most people believe the saying 'you are what you eat'. We know that regularly overdoing it with fatty or sugary foods piles on the pounds, which makes us look and feel unhealthy – and that can be stressful.

Surprisingly, though, stress is rarely directly caused by food or drink on their own. However, there is no doubt that certain foods can trigger unpleasant conditions like hyperactivity, insomnia, migraines and indigestion, which will increase the likelihood of the sufferer being stressed.

But people have to eat and drink to survive. Food and drink sustains them, providing energy and nutrients designed to keep mind and body in mint condition. Some foods are especially helpful, for example, in fighting infection or promoting the growth of strong bones.

It is essential, therefore, that you eat the right balance of foods. And, as no single food can provide all the nutrients you need – or actively reduce your stress as such – a healthy diet is one that is as varied as possible.

How healthy is your diet?

Find out by circling whichever number applies in each question and adding up your score:

	Never	Rarely	Sometimes	Often	Always
'I eat salty foods'	1	2	3	4	5
'I eat less than 5 portions of fruit and veg each day'	1	2	3	4	5
'I drink more than 3 units of alcohol each day'	1	2	3	4	5
'I eat/cook with butter'	1	2	3	4	5
'I drink less than 1.2 litres of fluid per day'	1	2	3	4	5
'I eat cakes and pastries'	1	2	3	4	5
'I add salt to my meals'	1	2	3	4	5
'I add sugar to hot drinks'	1	2	3	4	5
'I eat fried foods'	1	2	3	4	5
'I have sugary carbonated drinks'	1	2	3	4	5
'I leave excess fat on meat or skin on poultry'	1	2	3	4	5

Your score

The higher your score, the unhealthier your diet! The rest of this chapter is devoted to showing you how to make the changes you need in order to eat (and cook) more healthily.

A healthy diet can help

- Enhance your general well-being.
- Maintain the right weight for your gender, age, height and frame.
- Reduce the risk of diseases like heart disease, strokes, cancer, osteoporosis and diabetes.
- Provide the right nutrients, vitamins, minerals and fibre for optimum mental and physical health.

FOOD AND STRESS

When the going gets tough, the stressed reach for chocolate. There's nothing new about comfort eating. Most people have turned to sugary or starchy foods for temporary relief – but have you ever wondered why?

Our old friend, the fight or flight response, is largely to blame. In stressful situations the brain needs a quick supply of fuel to help it think and act quickly. Appetite (not deemed a priority) is temporarily suppressed and, because the brain cannot burn fat or proteins directly, the hormone cortisol stimulates the conversion of protein into glucose (a carbohydrate).

Stress increases the production of adrenaline which inhibits production of insulin but stimulates production of glucagon. These changes elevate blood glucose, fuelling the brain. Other hormones help sustain your blood volume and blood pressure – helpful if you lose body fluid through bleeding or sweating!

Some experts believe that diets high in refined sugars (biscuits, cakes) and stimulants (caffeine), or low in protein or fat could negatively affect the way people cope with stress. Sugar dips, for example (see page 147) are a common by-product of snacking on sweet foods.

ENSURING A BALANCED DIET

Recommendations for healthy eating are contained in the Government's *Balance of Good Health*. To maintain optimum health, people need to eat a variety of foods from Groups 1–4, which will provide most of your nutrients, and eat sparingly from Group 5. These five food groups comprise:

Group 1: Bread, other cereals and potatoes.
Group 2: Fruit and vegetables.
Group 3: Meat, fish and alternatives (including nuts and eggs).
Group 4: Milk and dairy foods.
Group 5: Foods containing fat and sugar – you need to limit your intake of foods from this group.

These apply for most people over the age of five. The food groups are explained in more detail overleaf.

The food groups....	How much can I have?
Bread, cereals and potatoes – includes bread, potatoes (and low fat oven chips), plantains, sweet potatoes, yams, pasta, breakfast cereals, oats, rice, noodles, millet, maize and cornmeal.	These should comprise a third of your daily food intake. Try to include one or more in each meal, (especially the wholegrain varieties). As a result, you'll eat less fat and more fibre.
Fruit and vegetables – these can be fresh, frozen, dried, canned or juiced. Beans (baked beans) and pulses (lentils and chickpeas) also count towards your 5-a-day.	Eat five or more 80g portions (e.g. a medium apple) daily. However much fruit juice and beans/ pulses you have, they only count towards one of your 5-a-day.
Meat, fish and alternatives – includes meat, poultry, fish (plus frozen and canned fish), eggs and alternatives (nuts, tofu, mycoprotein, textured vegetable protein, beans and pulses.	Some products (like sausages or beefburgers) can be high in fat, so eat these types of foods only occasionally, choosing low fat varieties wherever possible.
Milk and dairy – includes milk, cheese, yogurt, fromage frais as well as calcium fortified soya alternatives to milk.	Eat 2–3 servings (i.e. a 200ml glass of milk, or 30g cheese) a day. Choose lower fat versions as much as possible.
Foods with fat (cooking oils, all spreading fats, mayonnaise, cream, fried foods, crisps, chocolate, biscuits, puddings, ice-cream, cakes) and **sugar** (soft drinks, jam, sweets, cakes, pastries, puddings, ice cream, etc).	Some fat in your diet is essential but try to limit your intake of these foods, choosing low fat or reduced sugar varieties wherever possible. Do try not to add extra fat or sugar when cooking.

How you can eat more healthily

Eat a wide variety of foods.
Be active, eating the right amount to maintain a healthy weight.
Eat more starchy foods such as bread, cereals, pasta, potatoes and rice, choosing wholegrain varieties as much as possible.
Try to eat at least five portions of fresh, frozen, canned and juiced fruit and vegetables each day (see opposite page).
Cut down on foods high in saturated fat (like cream, pastry, lard).
Aim for no more than 6g of salt a day.
Avoid too many sugary foods and drinks.
Drink alcohol sensibly – current guidelines recommend no more than 2–3 units for women and 3–4 units for men per day. A unit is a pub measure of spirits, 125ml of wine or half a pint of beer.
Stick to regular meal-times and eat breakfast. Skipping meals can lead to bingeing on fatty or sugary foods.
Cut down on cigarettes.
Drink plenty of water – even being only slightly dehydrated affects performance and concentration.
Include more fish, especially oily fish like salmon or mackerel.
Enjoy your food!

TIP: Try relaxing with a cup of tea. This can be your usual brand or you can try something different – decaffeinated, herbal or fruit tea or decaffeinated green tea – for a change.

WHAT TO AVOID

Unfortunately, there are no foods or drinks that are specific stress-busters, but some people find that certain ones can actually trigger a variety of problems, such as:

- Headaches.
- Heartburn.
- Hyperactivity (in some people).
- Indigestion.
- Insomnia.
- Migraine.

Of course, everyone's different – so what causes problems for one person won't always affect another. Be more aware of what causes problems for you and, to maintain optimum health, try to minimize your intake of the following:

- Rich and fatty food.
- Some additives and preservatives (including colourings and flavourings).
- Carbonated drinks.
- Alcohol.
- Sugar/sugary foods.
- Tea, coffee, cola, chocolate, as well as energy drinks.

HEALTHY WAYS TO COOK

Somehow people seem to have lost the knack of cooking nowadays. Lack of time is the excuse, as they reach for the frying pan, slip another ready meal into the microwave or phone for a pizza.

Fast food has affected our palates too. Much of it contains high levels of fat, salt or sugar. Never mind the taste though, or any negative effect it may have on the body – a lot of of the appeal lies in the fact that it's available for consumption here and now.

The best way to reverse this unhealthy trend is to cook for yourself. This may mean devoting more time to shopping and preparing food. But it's worth it because you'll be better able to control the ingredients and produce more balanced meals.

There's no excuse not to. Bookshops are overflowing with easy-to-follow guides on how to cook, the television serves up a daily diet of cooking programmes, while modern equipment designed to facilitate the culinary endeavours of the general public is readily available.

The tips on the opposite page should help you in your quest for healthier cooking:

Healthier cooking

Microwave or steam rather than boil. Steaming preserves nutrients, particularly in vegetables, that are often lost in boiling. Steamed vegetables are pleasantly crunchy and somehow taste fresher.

Grill or bake rather than fry. Modern grill pans have grooves to capture the fat. If you do fry, *dry* fry, or use vegetable oils or polyunsaturated margarine instead of butter. Always trim excess fat off meat and remove the skin from poultry.

Include salad, uncooked and cooked vegetables in your meals. Broccoli, spinach and cabbage are delicious eaten raw and contain vital nutrients like vitamin C (see page 149).

Eat fish at least twice a week, including one portion of oily fish (like salmon or mackerel). This contains essential fatty acids which, studies have shown, can help improve the health of your heart and the condition of your skin.

Juicing is a great way to make up your five daily portions of fruit and vegetables. Remember though, servings of fruit juice can only count as one of your 5-a-day, no matter how much you drink. You can make juice from most fruits or vegetables (apart from bananas and avocadoes). Blueberries and strawberries especially contain antioxidants which may protect against cancer and heart disease.

Eat more brightly coloured vegetables, such as tomatoes, carrots and red, green and yellow peppers. These vegetables' phytochemicals may protect against disease.

EATING TO BEAT HIGH BLOOD PRESSURE

According to the Food Standards Agency (FSA), a third of people in the UK have high blood pressure, described as 'the force of blood pressing against the walls of the arteries as the heart pumps blood around the body.' Those with high blood pressure (also known as hypertension) are three times more likely to develop raised cholesterol and are also more at risk from heart disease, stroke or heart failure than those with normal blood pressure.

Many people believe that stress is a major cause. Undoubtedly your blood pressure goes up when you're stressed as a result of the fight or flight response. But this is temporary and usually goes back down when that stress has gone. The Blood Pressure Association (BPA) says there's no evidence that longer-term stress causes hypertension. Other factors, such as drinking too much alcohol, eating too much salt or overindulging in fatty or sugary foods, not taking enough exercise and becoming overweight – as well as a genetic predisposition – are far more significant causes of high blood pressure.

Salt plays an important role in the onset of high blood pressure. Too much can lead to fluid retention, meaning (in very simplistic terms) that the heart has to pump harder to push more fluid through the veins and arteries.

It's a good idea to limit your salt intake anyway. According to Consensus Action on Salt and Health (CASH), a group of specialists concerned with the effects of salt on health, excess salt is linked to osteoporosis (thinning of the bones), asthma, kidney disease and stomach cancer. Unfortunately, the main source of the UK's salt intake – around 75% to 80% – is hidden and therefore unconsciously consumed. That's because it is added to the manufacture and processing of food, including many products aimed at children.

Statistics from CASH show that stroke, heart failure and coronary heart disease are the UK's biggest killers, accounting for just under half of all deaths.

Research suggests however that 35,000 of the UK's stroke deaths could be saved each year if people reduced their salt intake by 3g per day.

If you think you may have high blood pressure, see your GP immediately. The good news is it can be treated – by medication, as well as by exercising and watching what you eat and drink.

Try the following

- Reduce your salt intake to less than 6g a day (less for children).
- Read food labels carefully. Look for the salt or

sodium figure per 100g. For example, 1.25g or more of salt per 100g or 0.5g of sodium or more per 100g is high, but 0.25g of salt or 0.1g of sodium per 100g is low.

- Don't add salt to food on the plate or when cooking. Increase flavour by adding garlic, chillies, lemon juice, herbs (like mint or coriander) or spices like pepper.

Avoid too much of the following:

Foods preserved in brine (salty water). For example, opt for tuna in spring water instead.

Processed food like salami, sausages, ham or bacon.

Salty and savoury snacks like crisps or salted nuts.

Table sauces like tomato ketchup or soy sauce.

Foods like cheese, bread and breakfast cereals are high in salt. Some cereals, for example, provide as much salt as Atlantic sea water! You should eat these foods as part of a balanced diet but try alternatives like cottage cheese, porridge oats and low-salt bread (available from many supermarkets and health food shops).

Use low-salt stock cubes or gravy powder (available from health food shops).

Eating more fruit and vegetables (a good source of potassium) can help lower blood pressure.

Keep your alcohol intake within recommended levels (see page 139).

IMPROVING DIGESTION

Digestion is the process by which food is broken down and used to provide energy and nutrients for growth and repair. It takes place in the nine-metre-long gastro-intestinal tract (including organs like the stomach or colon) that runs from the mouth to the anus.

Food is broken down into smaller particles by acid and enzymes in the small intestine. Rhythmic contractions and relaxations, called peristalsis, moves the food along. Peristalsis speeds up or slows down depending on the person's health and state of relaxation.

An important part of the process is the absorption of liquids through the wall of the colon into the bloodstream. Indigestible food progresses through the colon, getting drier until it's expelled via the anus. Food takes about 30 hours to go through the body – less with diarrhoea and more (up to 60 hours) with constipation. Around 3 million people in the UK regularly suffer with constipation – peristalsis slows down so more water is absorbed into the body, leaving hard, dry stools that are painful to expel.

The digestive tract is easily upset, the biggest culprits being fast foods, tension, hurried eating and lack of regular exercise.

Observing the following advice could help improve your digestion:

- Have three moderate-sized meals each day, supplemented with healthy snacks.
- Eat a fibre-rich diet (including plenty of fruit, vegetables, wholegrain bread and pasta, brown rice, wholegrain cereals, lentils) each day. This provides vital bulk to help food and waste products move along the tract more easily.
- Drink plenty of fluids– around at least 1.2 litres a day – to keep skin hydrated and flush out toxins. Not enough can lead to constipation.
- Always chew slowly and don't eat when angry or upset.
- Eat sitting down – eating on the go is often hurried and it's easy to lose track of the calories!
- Supplement with probiotics if necessary. Our large intestine normally has millions of 'feel-good' bacteria which help break down fibre. Sometimes these are destroyed by ill-health, poor diet or antibiotics and can be topped up via foods such as live yoghurt or probiotic drinks (available from health food shops or chemists).

TIP: If you don't like tap water, try filtering it. Tabletop and slimline fridge jugs are readily available from supermarkets and chemists. Keep jugs clean and change filters regularly.

CONTROLLING BLOOD SUGAR LEVELS

People who are stressed often don't eat regularly because the fight or flight response can suppress appetite. Irregular eating causes a drop in the body's blood sugar level which can lead to tiredness, irritability, poor concentration and anxiety. Even if you do eat regularly, these dips can occur naturally – often in the mid-morning or mid-afternoon.

Coping with a sugar dip

Avoid eating too many sugary foods and drinks. These release sugar quickly into the blood causing a peak in energy. But the body has to produce extra insulin to cope with the sugar, resulting in another sugar dip – and you're back to square one!

Eat a good breakfast, preferably including breakfast cereals or wholegrain toast. These types of foods take longer to digest and release energy slowly.

Keep healthy snacks like carrot sticks, fresh fruit, dried apricots or seeds handy.

If you're diabetic you'll probably already be managing your condition under medical supervision. If you suspect you may have diabetes, consult your GP urgently. Symptoms include increased thirst, a need to pass urine more often, especially at night, weight loss, tiredness, blurred vision and genital itching.

VITAMINS AND MINERALS

Despite being present in very small quantities, vitamins and minerals are essential for good health. There are two types of vitamins – fat-soluble and water-soluble. The fat-soluble variety – such as Vitamins A, D, E and K – are found in fatty and oily foods. The body stores these in the liver and fatty tissues so daily consumption isn't always necessary and too much can be harmful.

Water-soluble vitamins (such as Vitamins B6, B12 or C) are not stored in the body, so foods containing these vitamins are needed regularly. Many fruit and vegetables are a good source of Vitamin C, which is easily destroyed by exposure to the air, sunlight or in cooking. Minerals, like iron, calcium, sodium and magnesium, are important, as they help turn food into energy and build strong bones and teeth.

If you are following a balanced diet, you should be getting all your nutrients. If you decide to take supplements, check with your GP or pharmacist, as an excess of certain vitamins can be harmful. Pregnant women should avoid too much Vitamin A, for example, as it can harm their unborn baby. All women who may become pregnant should take a daily 400 microgram (mcg) folic acid supplement to help prevent neural tube defects like spina bifida.

Vitamin/ mineral	Function	Found in
Vitamin A (retinol)	Helps maintain vision in poor light, strengthens the immune system and maintains healthy skin and mucus linings (e.g. in the nose).	Liver, eggs, cheese, fish (mackerel), milk yoghurt.
Vitamin B6 (pyridoxine)	Enables the body to use and store energy from food and helps form haemoglobin (carries oxygen around the body).	Poultry, pork, bread, cereals, milk, potatoe soya.
Vitamin B12	Good for keeping the nervous system healthy and blood red, helps release energy from food.	Meat, cod, salmon, cheese, eggs, milk, yeast extract.
Vitamin C (ascorbic acid)	Helps the immune system by keeping cells healthy and assists in the absorption of iron from food.	Fruit and vegetables especially sweet potatoes, broccoli, oranges, kiwi fruit.
Calcium	Helps maintain bones, teeth and muscle fitness.	Milk, yoghurt, cheese, such as sardines, nuts
ron	Helps make red blood cells which transport oxygen around the body.	Lean red meat, liver, b nuts, cereals, dark gre leafy vegetables.
HA – the Omega-3 fatty cid	Helps maintain a healthy heart and plays a role in brain development.	Oily fish, fish oil supplements, Omega enriched eggs, some algae supplements.

THE ROLE OF DIETS

There's so much pressure to look good nowadays. Some people are constantly on weight loss diets – whether they need to be or not. Many diets restrict the intake of important foods – those containing carbohydrate or protein for example, which can affect digestion and reduce levels of vitamins, minerals and other important nutrients.

There are others, too, whose unhealthy eating habits are undermining their health and that of their children, who grow up to believe that fast foods and carbonated drinks are the only way to eat.

Being a healthy weight is important, of course. You look better, there's less strain on your joints and there's less risk of diabetes or heart disease.
But if you eat a balanced diet, restricting your intake of sugar, fat and salt and exercise moderately, there's no reason why you should have a weight problem.

Attention Deficit Hyperactivity Disorder (ADHD)

The term ADHD is used to describe people (usually children) with three main kinds of problems:

- overactive behaviour (hyperactivity)
- impulsive behaviour

- difficulty in paying attention (also called Attention Deficit Disorder, as sufferers aren't always hyperactive)

ADHD is a stressful condition for sufferers and their families. It can cause significant problems at school and make getting on with other children difficult. Families affected by ADHD need a lot of help and support. It is believed that this condition (affecting about 5 per cent of the UK's children and teenagers) can be exacerbated by sensitivity to foods containing additives and/or sugar.

Research has shown that the Feingold diet (eliminating food and drinks containing artificial colours, flavourings, preservatives and salicylates – chemicals found in some plants) may help manage symptoms in some children. But other factors, like exercise, rest and paying attention to overall health and nutrition are also important.

In some studies, sufferers have been found to have lower levels of essential fatty acids (EFAs) than other children. It is thought that giving them omega-3 and omega-6 fatty acid supplements may help their concentration and behaviour. Rich sources of omega 3 EFAs are oily fish like mackerel, herring or salmon and rich sources of omega-6 fatty acids are soya beans, walnuts, olives, sunflowers, corn and evening primrose oils.

FEEL BETTER NOW?

Are your eating habits any healthier? Try the quiz below:

Each day do you have....	Yes	No
1) Five portions of fruit and vegetables?		
2) Uncooked vegetables or salad?		
3) 6g of salt or less?		
4) Three portions of fibre-rich foods?		
5) Polyunsaturated low-fat spread?		
6) Breakfast?		
7) At least 1.2 litres of fluids?		
8) Less than two caffeinated drinks?		
9) One portion of oily fish each week?		
10) Have a home-cooked meal four times a week.		
Your total (score one point per 'yes' answer)		

Your score

8–10 points – Well done – keep up the good work!

5–7 points – Overall, you're doing well. Now focus on areas where you scored less well.

4 points or less – A poor diet can undermine your physical and mental health. If you're still concerned about your diet, consult your local GP. The British Nutrition Foundation website (see page 186) can help you find a dietician.

5-MINUTE FIXES: SLEEP

The sixteenth century poet Sir Philip Sidney described sleep as: *'the certain knot of peace...the balm of woe, the poor man's wealth, the prisoner's release...'* Most people would agree that a refreshing sleep is priceless – a necessary and welcome end to a tiring day and a restorative for body and soul alike. But Sir Philip was speaking five hundred years ago. Today's hectic modern lifestyle demands a lot of people, both physically and mentally.

What is sleep?

Sleep is a time when people stop perceiving the outside world. Most (Western) adults average 7.5 hours a night. There's no hard and fast rule, though, as people's needs differ. The elderly sleep less than, say, babies, usually because sleep is interrupted by, for example, arthritic pain or the need for the toilet.

Sleep occurs in several stages – light sleep, REM (rapid eye movement) when we experience dreaming, deeper sleep and very deep sleep when our brainwaves slow right down. Most people sleep deeply for 25% of the night, 50% is spent in light sleep and 25% in REM – usually at regular 90 minute intervals.

Why sleeping well is important

While you are sleeping...

...your muscles rest and recuperate. During the night when you're deeply asleep the body produces growth hormones that aid the healing process and help stimulate the immune system. Your brain remains busy (each night the body uses only 120 fewer calories to function than it did during the day), although activity slows during deep sleep. You dream, processing all that you've experienced during the day.

Why sleep problems occur

There are many causes of insomnia (problems getting to or staying asleep) including simple things like being too hot or cold. Young children, medication and painful conditions like arthritis can also cause wakefulness – as can anxiety. Sleeplessness can persist even when the original cause is removed, becoming established as a pattern of behaviour. The more you worry about it, the worse it gets. Insomnia can result in the following:

- Poor concentration
- Daytime sleepiness
- Being accident prone
- Fatigue
- Forgetfulness
- Irritability

PREPARING FOR TOMORROW BEFORE SLEEPING

The unfinished business of the day can prey on your mind, causing sleeplessness. So make sure you complete your day before going to bed. As well as helping to avoid an unnecessary and stressful rush the next morning, getting ready the night before can also help you wind down. The following tasks should only take 10 minutes or so and could include:

- Emptying the dishwasher and putting everything away.
- Ensuring the kitchen is tidy and laying the table for tomorrow's breakfast.
- Filling the kettle.
- Packing your briefcase/the children's schoolbags.
- Packing your/the children's lunchboxes and putting them in the fridge overnight.
- Laying out your clothes and cleaning your shoes.
- Checking your calendar or diary for what's happening tomorrow.
- Making a brief list of things you have to do the next day.

TIP: Putting packed bags and anything else that you might need for the next day near the door ready to go will minimize the chance that you might forget something important!

ORGANIZING YOUR BEDROOM

Your bedroom should be a haven of peace and tranquillity, away from the hustle and bustle of daily life. However, if the debris of your life has set up camp in your bedroom, that could be one reason why you aren't sleeping as well as you should.

Getting organized in your bedroom
Keep your bedroom clean and well aired. Getting rid of dust can help reduce sneezing and asthmatic coughing if you are sensitive to dust mites.
Be tidy. There's nothing worse than opening your bedroom door to a muddle. Clutter is also stressful, according to Feng Shui experts, because it blocks the chi, the vital energy force that normally flows everywhere (see Chapter 8). We're at our most vulnerable when we sleep, exposed to the forces and energies around us. The chi should be able to flow everywhere, including under our beds, so we awake fully refreshed.
Organize your bedroom so everything is stored away in cupboards and drawers to allow the chi to flow freely. Keep surfaces (like window sills and bedside tables) as clear as possible. This also helps reduce the build-up of dust.

SOOTHING LIGHTING

Turning down the lights in your living room and bedroom at night creates a soothing, relaxing atmosphere that helps get you and your family in the mood for sleep. Your bedroom is your sanctuary. You have cleaned, tidied and organized it and all the clutter has gone. It's now time to make it soothing. Here's how you can do this:

Avoid harsh high wattage bulbs in your bedroom and use soft pearl bulbs in a lower wattage instead.

Invest in a couple of dimmer switches for your bedroom and living room. During the evening turn these down to make your living room restful and prepare you for bedtime.

Place lamps around your bedroom and living room that reflect a soft glow onto your walls – which are preferably a neutral or soothing colour.

Cover up the harsh glow of alarm clock LEDs before you go to sleep so that they will not disturb you if you should turn towards them during the night.

Harness your own body clock by choosing light curtains for your bedroom. In the morning these will let in light and awaken you naturally – much kinder to your body than the harsh buzz of your alarm clock!

AROMATHERAPY

Aromatherapy is the use of concentrated essential oils extracted from flowers, herbs, trees, woods, seeds, leaves and fruits. The art of aromatherapy is an ancient one, regularly used by the Egyptians, Indians and Chinese. Modern aromatherapy was invented in 1928 by Rene-Maurice Gattefosse, a French chemist. Many medical experts agree that essential oils can be beneficial in relieving stress and related health problems. They are used by the National Health Service, for example, in midwifery and in the care of cancer patients.

Use of aromatherapy

Aromatherapy oils can be stimulating, uplifting or soothing. Frequently used in massage, the oils can also be put in baths as well as burners or candles to allow the scent to flow freely throughout the room. If inhaled, the oils enter the bloodstream via the lungs which contain blood capillaries. Or they go through the olfactory nerves (in the nose) into the brain, which interprets the smell. The limbic system (which is the part of the brain responsible for our memory and emotions) takes over and allows us to create or retrieve memories associated with smell. Aromatherapy oils are very effective in massage, too.

The main aromatherapy stressbusters

- **Cleansing/uplifting/stimulating**
  Bergamot
  Cypress
  Juniper

- **Calming/relaxing/soothing/balancing**
  Chamomile
  Marjoram
  Geranium
  Lavender
  Mandarin
  Grapefruit
  Neroli (is good for panic attacks)
  Rose (is very nurturing, especially for the female reproductive system)

- **Grounding**
  Frankincense
  Sandalwood

How to use aromatherapy oils

- The essential oils are highly volatile and must be kept in dark glass bottles, even when blended. Any oils or products in clear glass or plastic containers will not be real aromatherapy.
- They are toxic substances, so do not drink them!

- Avoid certain oils if you are pregnant.
- Keep out of the eyes and use only lavender or tea tree neat on the skin.
- Be careful when buying oils, as some are not the true essence.
- Consult a qualified aromatherapist (make sure they're on the Aromatherapy Council's register). This can be cheaper than buying the oils yourself and often the first consultation will be free. If in doubt, check with your doctor first.

Bathing with aromatherapy oils

What better end to a long, hard day than a relaxing soak in a warm aromatherapy bath? In fact, bathing is one of the best ways to experience essential oils because you inhale them and absorb them through the skin.

- For a relaxing bath add up to 10 drops of essential oil (such as lavender or chamomile) to the bath and agitate to mix properly.
- Don't have the bath too hot as you might feel faint or sick.
- Just lie and soak for 20 minutes, without washing as your soap will interfere with the action of the oils.
- If you don't want to use essential oils, a wide range of aromatherapy-based soap, bath minerals and other bath products is also freely available, but buy from an aromatherapy supplier to make sure it is from a botanical source.

AROMATHERAPY CANDLES

Candles made with essential oils can create an uplifting, refreshing or soothing feel to the room. During the evening, though, when your thoughts are turning towards sleep, calming fragrances such as lavender, rose or mandarin are best.

Aromatherapy candles come in all shapes and sizes. There are pillar, taper or tea light candles plus candles in tins and jars.

Many are made from organic essential oils, free from artificial dyes and perfumes that can cause allergies. Beeswax and pure soybean wax candles are an increasingly popular alternative to the traditional paraffin variety. Aromatherapy candles are freely available both online and in shops.

Essential oils can also be diffused via:

- Essential oil burners – several drops of the essential oil are put into a small bowl of water which is heated by a tea light.
- Boiling water – the oils are put direct into boiling water which avoids the potential fire hazard.
- Light bulb rings – these use the heat from light bulbs.
- Fan diffusers – these blow air over a tray or pad of oil and are a very effective means of diffusion.

RELAXING WITH HERBS

Herbs have been used since ancient times to relieve a wide variety of conditions – and are the basis for many modern medicines. Some, like chamomile, limeflower and lavender flower, have a calming and relaxant effect that can help you unwind.

How to use herbs

- Pour boiling water on herbs or teabags containing the herbs (teabags are available from supermarkets and health food shops) and infuse for 5–10 minutes for a natural alternative to caffeinated drinks.
- Take 10–15 drops of *Valeriana officinalis* (available from herbalists or health food shops) an hour before going to bed.
- A cup of tea made with lavender flowers can relieve a stress headache. Put a tablespoon onto some lint or bandage, apply this to your forehead and sit quietly for ten minutes. You can drink the rest of the tea afterwards.
- For a nervous stomach and nausea caused by stress, mix equal parts of peppermint leaves with Chamomile flowers (use a teaspoon to a mug of hot water) and infuse for 5–10 minutes. Sip while hot.
- Do consult a practitioner from the National Institute of Medical Herbalists (details on page 187) if you are pregnant, breastfeeding, or taking prescribed drugs.

BEATING INSOMNIA

The following might help if you are still having trouble sleeping:

Re-programme your body clock by going to bed and getting up at the same time every day, including weekends and holidays.

Keep the bedroom comfortable and restful:

- Use the bedroom for sleep and sex only. So no reading, eating, watching TV or working there!
- Maintain the right temperature – not too hot or too cold.
- Keep your bedroom well-aired.
- Invest in good quality pillows and mattresses for comfort.
- Keep your bedroom tidy and free of clutter.
- Minimize unwanted light if that's a problem, using dark curtains, black-out blinds or an eye mask.

Minimize noise.

- Ask noisy neighbours (politely) to turn down their television or radio late at night (or contact the relevant council department if necessary).
- Invest in some ear plugs, available from all good chemists.
- Consider buying an inexpensive white-noise machine to block unwanted sounds, unless you have young children, in which case you will need to be more alert.

See your doctor if you're in pain, and your regular painkillers aren't helping.

Take regular exercise. If you're active, you're more likely to enjoy a deeper and more refreshing sleep. Try to avoid exercising too close to bedtime.

Don't go to bed hungry but don't overeat either.

- Avoid alcohol and caffeine (including coffee, tea, cola and chocolate) for six hours before turning in.
- If you're hungry, eat a light snack of healthy food like carrots or drink skimmed milk.
- Don't drink too many liquids, or you will need the toilet during the night.

Don't actively *try* to sleep as this causes anxiety.

If you're wakeful, get out of bed for 15–30 minutes, read a non-stimulating book or do something boring, returning only when sleepy.

Relax - if necessary visualize yourself relaxing somewhere nice, on the beach, under a tree – anywhere.

- Try to avoid looking at your bedside clock.
- Keep a notebook beside your bed to write down any thoughts. This stops you fidgeting that you'll forget something important.

If you're experiencing emotional pain (like relationship difficulties or a relationship breakdown), talk it over with a counsellor or someone you trust. Bottling up unresolved issues definitely does not promote healthy sleep and can be detrimental to your overall health in the long run.

Establish a relaxing bedtime routine that works for you and stick to it.

FEEL BETTER NOW?

It helps to have a relaxing bedtime routine. Do you have one?

Is your bedroom calm and relaxed? (pages 157–8)
Are your organised for the next day? (page 156)
Have you had a relaxing aromatherapy bath? (page 161)
Have you used any herbal remedies? (page 163)
Have you had a light bedtime snack? (page 165)
Have you done a visualization exercise? (page 50)

How are you feeling now? Score one point for each 'yes' answer:

	Yes	No
1) Do you sleep for between 6 and 9 hours?		
2) Do you wake up feeling refreshed?		
3) Are you more alert now?		
4) Are you less tense and irritable?		
5) Have you cut down on caffeine/alcohol?		
6) Do you exercise more?		
7) Is your bedroom calm and relaxed?		
8) Do you talk about your worries?		
Your total		

Your score
6–8 points – Your hard work has paid off! Keep it up.
4–7 points – You're on the right track.
3 points or less – Focus on one area, moving on when ready.

If you are still having problems, other options include:

Hypnosis

Hypnosis has been described as an altered mental state in which the brain is unfocussed and, under hypnosis people become calmer and more receptive to positive suggestion.

By programming correct information into the subconscious, hypnosis can make long-lasting changes to thoughts, feelings and behaviour.

Hypnosis can also:

- Lower anxiety.
- Lower blood pressure.
- Relax muscle tone.
- Ingrain positive suggestion.
- Make you sleep more quickly and deeply. Always consult a qualified hypnotherapist (see page 189 for the British Society for Medical & Dental Hypnosis' website details).

Your GP

He or she can check for any biological causes (such as thyroid disorders or depression), and suggest some alternative sleep remedies. If your problems persist your GP may refer you to one of several UK specialist sleep centres.

LONGER TERM SOLUTIONS

Stress is incredibly difficult to avoid, since the causes of it are, literally, everywhere! The last few chapters have been devoted to showing you how to cope with it more effectively. I've referred to many of these stress-busters – exercising, massage, aromatherapy baths and so on – as '5-minute fixes' – because they are relatively easy changes to make. But even 5-minute fixes need repeating regularly if they are to make a lasting difference to your life.

Not all methods of stress reduction are so straightforward. It's important to remember that your reaction determines whether the outcome of a stressful event is positive or negative. So, to quote Dr Chris Johnstone, the author of *Find Your Power*: *'10 per cent of life is what happens and 90% about how you respond.'*

Some events, like the death of a loved one, are truly devastating and you can't control those. But so many causes of stress originate from within – and those can be controlled – at least if you know how.

Taking control means changing the way you think and behave – and that can involve a long and difficult journey of self-discovery. But it's one that will be well worth it in the end.

FINDING THE NEW YOU!

To manage stress positively, you must think differently about your life and what causes you difficulty. You can do this in several ways:

Neuro-linguistic programming (NLP)

Neuro-Linguistic Programming (NLP) studies the structure of how humans think and experience the world. People derive their outlook from how they filter and perceive information gained via their senses from the world around, and behave accordingly. Repeating old unhelpful behaviour patterns with negative results is a major cause of stress. NLP can help you make sense of the world and create opportunities for personal change.

Positive thinking

Studies show that thinking positively can help lower stress and improve your well-being.

- Work on turning negative thoughts into positive ones. Think about what you are saying to yourself. Would you say such things to anyone else?
- Regard new tasks as opportunities to learn a new skill and further your personal development.
- Worried about time pressure? Delegate, prioritize and say no to other commitments (see page 171).
- Don't be afraid to ask others for help – two heads are often better than one!

Embrace your inner strength

Life's many challenges can be extremely stressful. But it's how you deal with the stress that counts. Do you avoid it? Doing so regularly could mean you have 'shrinking life syndrome' – you're at the mercy of your fears because you haven't faced them and you stop growing as a person. Facing our fears and stresses isn't easy. Overcoming them is even more difficult.

If you've ever triumphed over a seemingly impossible obstacle, you'll probably remember how strong you felt afterwards! Each victory strengthens you to face the next hurdle – and the next. But this requires harnessing your inner strength and resolve, by:

- Defining what you really want and drawing up a clear roadmap for getting there.
- Understanding how you look at life (see page 169) and identifying unhelpful behaviour patterns which must be changed so you can progress.
- Seeing failure as an inevitable part of life which can provide valuable lessons in how to succeed next time.
- Being more assertive (see page 169).
- Thinking more positively – see hurdles as opportunities to be embraced.
- Life is generally enjoyable, so be happy!

Being assertive

Are you scared to turn down extra tasks or 'put upon' by family and friends? Being more assertive could save a lot of angst, time and effort. Assertiveness is about having enough self-worth to understand that you have a right to enjoy your life. It's about drawing clear boundaries and communicating these calmly and respectfully. It's also about valuing the rights of others.

Assertiveness is not about

- Saying yes to keep the peace.
- Acting aggressively.
- Always getting your own way.
- Controlling others.

Being assertive
Use open body language (see chapter 3), standing up straight.
Make eye contact but don't stare (this can seem aggressive).
Always try to remain calm .
Be honest about your feelings, using 'I' language, e.g. 'I need'.
Be respectful and don't attack the other person's opinion.
Repeat your message if necessary, acknowledging that you've understood what they've said.
Try offering alternative solutions to satisfy you both.

MAKE TIME FOR YOURSELF

Stressed people never have time for themselves – usually because they're not assertive enough. They're so busy looking after the needs of others that their own requirement for time and space gets forgotten.

Does this sound like you? Everyone deserves some time to themselves – and that includes you, so don't feel guilty. Besides, time out can be energizing, enabling you to pick up where you left off with renewed vigour. So, what are you going to do with your free time? Here are a few suggestions:

Having some 'Me' time
Pamper yourself with a relaxing soak in the bath, (see Chapter 7) or treat yourself to a massage (see Chapter 5).
Curl up and read a favourite book.
Record your thoughts in a diary.
Chill out in the garden with a long, cool drink and a magazine.
Go window shopping or treat yourself to those clothes or that CD you've got your eye on.
Go and see that new film, alone or with friends – it's up to you.
Do some exercise (see page 174) or lose yourself in your favourite hobby (see opposite).
Feeling better now? Good!

Cultivate a hobby

Make time for yourself – and lose yourself in something you really enjoy at the same time.

Some hobby ideas

Fancy learning a language? There are many books/ CDs/ DVDs and videos available to help you learn. Meet like-minded people by taking a course at your local adult education centre.

Creative writing can be a great outlet for your emotions. You may discover a side of you that you never knew existed. Check out your local adult education centre/telephone directory for courses.

What about gardening? You can combine your creative side with being outdoors – and enjoy the results every time you relax in your garden.

Can you draw or paint? Even if you can't, would you like to learn and explore your creative side?

How about learning to play a musical instrument? Music can profoundly affect your mood and provide an excellent way to release all those pent-up emotions. Perhaps you've already tried and given up because you didn't have the time to practise. Now's the time to make the time and there's no reason why you shouldn't find it really worthwhile.

Other ideas you could explore include wine-making,cake decorating and pottery.

Be more active

As you've seen in Chapter 3, regularly getting rid of physical tension can help lower your stress levels, your blood pressure and make you feel calmer. You'll see a difference in how you look as well as how you feel. And there are social benefits, too, in that you'll interact with like-minded people. So, if you haven't already decided which type of sport or exercise you'd like to try, rest assured that there are many different ones available to suit every taste and fitness level.

If you like being outdoors, walking, jogging, tennis, football or cycling can give you an excellent workout. Indoor activities include squash, dancing, badminton, weight training. You can give your mind a workout, too, via Yoga, Tai Chi or Pilates which combine carefully-controlled physical activity with breathing.

The choice is yours. But to realize the benefits any physical activity must be done regularly.

TIP: To find a local yoga, pilates, tai chi or fitness class click on www.bwy.org.uk/teachers/local_teachers.asp (yoga)
www.pilatesfoundation.com/locate.php
www.taichiunion.com/instructors.php
www.touchlocal.com/nat/c-989-th+Clubs+Fitness+Centres

Meditate for peace of mind

Meditating can soothe and calm the mind. Just withdrawing (temporarily) from the outside world and focusing your attention on your body can create a state of deep relaxation, allowing fatigue and stress to melt away.

Although meditation is an ancient art, modern studies show that it can help reduce blood pressure. Regular meditators are happier, healthier, more relaxed and more productive.

HOW TO MEDITATE

1) Choose a time and place free of interruptions. Be comfortable (warm, with loose clothing, etc.).
2) Sit or lie down comfortably.
3) Light a candle and/or play soothing music.
4) Close your eyes and breathe deeply, allowing air to flow into the lungs.
5) Create a safe place in your mind to allow your thoughts to run freely. Visualize a place where you were happy (see page 50).
6) Focus on your breathing and count your breaths from 1–10 (inhaling/exhaling counts as one breath), until the need to count dissolves.
7) Practise for 20 minutes, twice a day if possible. Meditation can be done almost anywhere.

GOLDEN BALL VISUAL MEDITATION

1) Sit comfortably. You can shut your eyes if you wish.
2) Hold your hands in front of you, level with your belly button. Imagine you're holding a golden ball.
3) With every out-breath that you make you are aiming to inflate the ball.

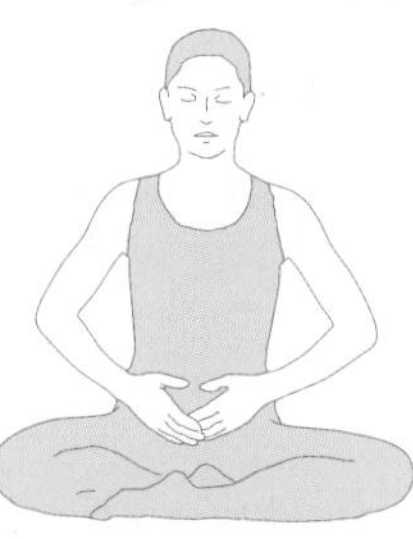

The 'golden ball' meditation exercise.

4) Notice how your warm breath feels inside the ball. How does the texture of the ball feel against your fingertips? How large is the ball now?
5) Fill in details as you wish. Are there colours, textures, sounds or feelings? Allow them to occur naturally.

Benefits of this exercise

- You have time and space away from the outside world.
- Focusing on this task and co-ordinating your breathing can really clear your mind.
- It helps lower your heart rate temporarily, which can be beneficial for your blood pressure.
- It can also be done in a public place. Camouflage it by putting your hands in your lap!

MAKE THE MOST OF FAMILY HOLIDAYS

Remember the old saying 'a change is as good as a rest'? Well, it's true! Getting away from it all, even for just a couple of days, can provide a welcome break from your usual routine and help recharge your batteries. You'll come back fully energized and refreshed, ready to throw yourself back into your life again.

By taking a holiday, you can also spend some quality time with your children, which they will appreciate just as much as you do. Going away for longer will give you the chance to unwind more completely, and you'll be able to feel the stress just melt away.

However, planning and going on holiday can be sources of anxiety in themselves, so here are some tips to help make the process easier:

- Think about what sort of holiday you'd like and discuss this with your family, including your children. This way you can plan activities that suit everyone.
- **Pets** – Organize their holiday care well in advance.
- **Holiday date** – Decide on a holiday date and put it into your diary immediately. Inform your employer (you will probably need permission to take a holiday anyway) and then nearer the time, you can delegate work, or ask your boss to take care of it.

- **Children** – Choose a holiday that has good family-friendly facilities and a playgroup or crèche that offers fun for your children – and gives you some peace for a couple of hours!
- **Passports** – If you're going abroad, check your passports in advance to ensure they haven't expired.
- **Budgeting** – Set yourself a budget and stick to it. Getting large credit card bills after you return calm and chilled from holiday will wind you up again. Try to get into the habit of saving each month towards the holiday, to ease the financial pain.
- **Vaccinations** – do you need these? Check in advance with your GP.
- **Insurance** – Despite the best-laid plans of mice and men… things can go wrong! So why not ease that worry by taking out some reasonably-priced insurance?
- **First aid** – Take a first aid kit with you, just in case. These are easily available from all good chemists.
- **Long journeys** – ease the boredom of long flights, car or train journeys by having plenty of favourite toys, colouring books, pens and puzzles for little travellers, and books and CDs for the adults.

TIP: If you're feeling exhausted, don't plan a busy city tour with early mornings and rigid timetables. Why not book a holiday where you can do some lazing about for a change?

Stress-free air travel

Some people find flying very stressful. Ensure that you are relaxed and comfortable when flying long distance by:

- Having a good night's sleep the night before flying.
- Eating a light meal beforehand.
- Drinking plenty of water before and during the flight. Try to avoid alcohol, as this can cause dehydration.
- Exercising your limbs gently, if you can (by circling your wrists and ankles) and try to walk around the plane at regular intervals.
- Wearing special socks (available from good chemists) to help reduce the risk of thrombosis during a long flight.

Driving comfortably

Here's how to ensure that your family holiday car journey is as relaxed as possible:

Plan your route well in advance, trying to avoid any congestion hotspots or roadworks.

Follow the advice (page 79) regarding posture when driving.

Take plenty of drinks, a flask of tea or coffee and some healthy snacks for you and the children.

Take frequent breaks to stretch your body and relax your eyes if you're driving a long way.

LIVE MORE SIMPLY

Your home should be a haven of peace and tranquillity, far away from the cares of the outside world. Try to make your rooms warm and inviting, as well as relaxing. Attractive décor and low lighting can help achieve this, as will only having the furniture you actually need. Too much will look cluttered (which is stressful) and it will prevent the free flow of life energy or *chi* (see opposite page).

Living a simpler life
Regularly weed out anything you don't use or wear any more. Recycle items that are in good condition by giving them to friends (e.g. baby clothes) or to charity.
Be firm with family and friends about what they bring into/and leave in your home. Teach your children that if they get out a toy or book, they must put it back in its rightful place after they've finished with it.
Be organized! File away paperwork, clearly labelling files so you can quickly retrieve information if necessary. Weed the files regularly, as paperwork can quickly pile up. Pay bills promptly and file away correspondence (or throw it away if you will not need it again).
Get yourself off junk mail and telephone lists via the mail preference service: http://www.mpsonline.org.uk/mpsr/ or telephone preference service: http://www.tpsonline.org.uk/tps/

Clear out clutter and promote good chi

Clutter absorbs the energy called *chi* which normally flows freely everywhere. According to the principles of Feng Shui, chi (also known as *shen chi*) is an invisible energy which sustains us and our environment. If chi is obstructed by clutter it can become trapped and stagnates. It then becomes a negative energy (described as *sha chi*) that draws in all other available energy including our own energy. What happens then is that we energize the room, rather than the room energizing us.

HOW TO ENSURE GOOD CHI

- Keep the front entrance to your house clear of clutter so the chi can flow in unhindered.
- Flat ceilings best promote the flow of chi. Avoid sleeping or working directly underneath exposed beams.
- Avoid overcrowding your house with furniture.
- Keep the toilet door closed and toilet lid down to slow the escape of chi, which can be attracted to water.
- In your kitchen, ensure that there is adequate space between the fridge, washing machine, sink and stove.
- Your lounge should be the heart of your home. Arrange furniture so that chi can gently flow around it.
- Open your bedroom windows for at least 30 minutes each day to allow fresh chi in.
- Keep your study or workroom free of clutter to enable the flow of chi and promote maximum creativity.

REVIEW YOUR KEY RELATIONSHIPS

Here's the $64,000 question: how are your family and friends reacting to the new you? Have they noticed any changes? If so, do they find you:

- calmer
- stronger
- more assertive
- positive
- focused
- relaxed
- more fun to be with?

If not, how else do they see you? How do they feel about the way you've altered? You may need to be careful here, because when people perceive any changes to their loved ones, this can cause them anxiety. Try to make the reasons why you're making changes to your life clear to them – and explain how they can help you. They've no doubt seen how stressed you've been, so they should understand your reasons – and be supportive.

You filled in a quiz on page 28 gauging the level of support that you receive from family and friends. Now that you've mastered our stress-busting techniques, become more assertive and harnessed your inner strength, have another go at it. How does it look now?

REVIEW YOUR JOB/CAREER

Remember the work stress questionnaire on page 24? Now that, hopefully, you are thinking more positively and have defined what you want out of life, why not have another go at it. How do the results look this time?

Do remember that you are more powerful than you think. So you can directly influence some aspects of your working life, such as:

- Your relationship with colleagues.
- Having adequate time to get your work done (try prioritizing), leaving work promptly and not taking work home (being assertive).

Even if you can't directly control certain aspects, you can influence the situation – often by being assertive.

- Be clear with your boss about what you can and can't do in the time given.
- Be clear about your career goals and request more training if necessary.
- If you're being bullied, keep a note of incidents and report these to your superior. Most organizations have a clear policy of how to deal with harassment. If the bully is your boss, talk to their superior or your human resources department.

FEEL BETTER NOW?

Do you remember the four questions on page 36? If you've still got your answers, have a look at them.

1) For question one, did you have any success when/if you tackled them? Could you have done anything differently? What can you do now?

2) For question 2, did you strike anything from your list? Did anyone notice? If they did, how did you deal with that? Could you have done anything differently? What can you do now?

3) If you're making time for yourself, the list in question 3 should be better balanced. If you find something draining, do you really have to do it? If so, what can you do to improve the situation? If it affects anyone else, how are you going to let them know. The section on assertiveness (page 171) should help you.

Finally, if you have goals you haven't yet realized, write down how you're going to get there – and focus!

You should be able to deal with stress more effectively now. As a reminder, check out the tips in the box opposite. If any particularly apply to you, make a note of these and keep them close to you at all times.

Long-term stress beaters

Get enough rest. If sleep is still a problem, re-read Chapter 7.

Relax regularly, using meditation, progressive muscle relaxation or whatever works for you.

Work off stress and anger with physical activity.

Look after yourself – by eating healthily, drinking plenty of fluid and avoiding excess caffeine, alcohol and tobacco.

Listen to your body. Rest if you're ill. Recognize the warning signs of stress, anger or anxiety and do what works for you.

Allow yourself guilt-free time to cultivate a hobby or pamper yourself.

Be assertive.

Be more organized and manage your time better.

Prioritize and stop doing things that don't benefit anyone.

Tackle one task at a time.

Delegate. If you just can't, then talk to your boss about getting some of your workload shifted.

Allow for the unexpected.

Spend time with people who help and support you (and for whom you do the same).

You can't always change things, so learn to accept them.

Have fun and laugh more!

If you're not getting any relief from your stress via the suggestions in this book, you should seek medical help. Your strress may be the symptom of an underlying condition that needs medical diagnosis/treatments to be treated. If there's nothing wrong, at least you'll get some reassurance!

USEFUL ADDRESSES

Aromatherapy Trade Council
P.O. Box 387
Ipswich
Suffolk IP2 9AN
Tel: 01473 603630
E-mail: info@a-t-c.org.uk
www.a-t-c.org.uk

Blood Pressure Association
60 Cranmer Terrace
London SW17 0QS
Tel: 020 8772 4994
http://www.bpassoc.org.uk/information/lifestyle/alcohol.htm

British Autogenic Society
The Royal London Homoeopathic Hospital
Great Ormond Street
London WC1N 3HR
Tel: 020 7391 8908
www.autogenic-therapy.org.uk

British Chiropractic Association
59 Castle Street
Reading
Berkshire RG1 7SN
Tel: 0118 950 5950
Email: enquiries@chiropractic-uk.co.uk
www.chiropractic-uk.co.uk

British Nutrition Foundation
High Holborn House
52 - 54 High Holborn
London, WCIV 6RQ
Tel: 020 7404 6504
www.nutrition.org.uk

British Osteopathic Association
Langham House West
Mill Street, Luton
Bedfordshire LU1 2NA
Tel: 01582 488455
Email: enquiries@osteopathy.org
www.osteopathy.org

British Wheel of Yoga
BWY Central Office
25 Jermyn Street
Sleaford
Lincolnshire NG34 7RU
Tel: 01529 306851
Email: office@bwy.org.uk
www.bwy.org.uk

General Council for Massage Therapy
27 Old Gloucester Street
London WC1N 3XX
Tel: 0870 8504452
Email: gcmt@btconnect.com
www.gcmt.org.uk

National Institute of Medical Herbalists
Elm House
54 Mary Arches Street
Exeter EX4 3BA
Tel: 01392 426022
Fax: 01392 498963
E-mail:
nimh@ukexeter.freeserve.co.uk
www.NIMH.org.uk

The Sleep Council
High Corn Mill, Chapel Hill
Skipton
North Yorkshire BD23 1NL
Tel: 01756 791089
Email: info@sleepcouncil.org.uk
www.sleepcouncil.org.uk

The Society of Teachers of the Alexander Technique
1st Floor, Linton House
39-51 Highgate Road
London NW5 1RS
Tel: 0845 230 7828
Fax: 020 7482 5435
Email: office@stat.org.uk
www.stat.org.uk

The Stress Management Society
PO Box 193
Harrow
Middlesex HA1 3ZE
Tel: 0870 199 3260
Email: info@stress.org.uk

USEFUL WEBSITES

What is stress?
Anxiety Coach – online guide to anxiety www.anxietycoach.com
British Heart Foundation www.bhf.org.uk
Health & Safety Executive www.hse.gov.uk
International Stress Management Association (ISMA) www.isma.org.uk
Dr Chris Johnstone www.chrisjohnstone.info
Mind www.mind.org.uk
Mood gym – a free online emotional self-help programme http://moodgym.anu.edu.au
Online information about stress stressbusting.co.uk
Science Museum www.sciencemuseum.org.uk/nakedscience/stress)

5-minute fixes: The body
Alexander Technique practitioner Stephanie Smith's website www.thealexanderpractice.co.uk

5-minute fixes: Breathing

British Thoracic Society
www.brit-thoracic.org.uk

5-minute fixes: Stretching and Massage

Scottish Massage Schools and Massage Therapists Organisation
www.scotmass.co.uk

5-minute fixes: Eating

British Hypertension Society
www.bhsoc.org

Food Standards Agency
www.foodstandards.gov.uk
www.eatwell.gov.uk

Mental Health Foundation
www.mentalhealth.org.uk

5-minute fixes: Sleep

British Society of Medical & Dental Hypnosis
www.dsmdh.org

Dr Andre Hedger & Associates Dental Practice (using hypnosis)
www.openwide.biz

Longer term solutions

Balanced Approach
www.balancedapproach.co.uk
(www.kaiming.co.uk for Tai Chi information and classes)

Feng Shui Society
www.fengshuisociety.org.uk
(Raymond Catchpole: Feng Shui, 9 Ki & Vastu consultant. raymondcatchpole@btinternet.com)

Online life skills courses/self-help training programme
www.livinglifetothefull.com

Transcendental Meditation UK
www.t-m.org.ukBatmanghelidj,

FURTHER READING

Batmanghelidj, F, *Your Body's Many Cries for Water: A Revolutionary Natural Way to Prevent Illness and Restore Good Health* (Tagman Press, 2004)

Bradley, Dinah, *Self-Help for Hyperventilation Syndrome: Recognizing and Correcting Your Breathing-Pattern Disorder* (Hunter House Publishers, 2001)

Brown, Christina, *The Yoga Bible: The Definitive Guide to Yoga Postures* (Godsfield Press Ltd, 2003)

Brignell, Roger, *The Pilates Handbook* (Island Books, UK)

Diagram Group, *Gem Body Language* (Collins, 1999)

Diamond, Joan, *Understanding the Alexander Technique* (First Stone Publishing, 2003)

Friedeberger, Julie, *Office Yoga: Tackling Tension with Simple Stretches You Can Do at Your Desk* (Motilal Banarsidass, India, 1999)

Hale, Gill *The Feng Shui Garden* (Aurum Press, 1998)

Idzikowski, Dr Chris, *Need to Know? Sleep* (Collins, 2007)

Johnstone, Dr Chris, *Find Your Power – boost your inner strengths, break through blocks and achieve inspired action* (Nicholas Brealey Publishing, 2006)

Martin, Paul *The Sickening Mind: Brain, Behaviour, Immunity and Disease* (Flamingo, 1998)

Maxwell-Hudson, Clare, *The Complete Book of Massage* (Dorling Kindersley, 1988)

Robinson, Ronnie, *Gem Tai Chi* (Collins, 2001)

Roland, Paul, *Gem Meditation* (Collins, 2002)

Sharon, Michael, *Nutrients A-Z: A User's Guide to Foods, Herbs, Vitamins, Minerals and Supplements* (Carlton Books Ltd, 2005)

Stacey, Jenny, *Steam Cooking: 100 Delicious and Healthy Food Receipes for All Steamers* (Apple Press, 2001)

INDEX

ACKNOWLEDGEMENTS

The author would like to thank the following people for their kind assistance in compiling this book: Dr Chris Johnstone; Dr Chris Idzikowski; Dr James Hawkins; Dr Andre Hedger (British Society of Medical & Dental Hypnosis); Tabitha Evans (British Wheel of Yoga); Stephanie Smith (Society of the Teachers of the Alexander Technique); Mark Peters (Balanced Approach); Trudy Norris (National Institute of Medical Herbalists); Carole Preen (Aromatherapy Trade Council); Tammy Mindel (The British Autogenic Society); Anna Denny (British Nutrition Foundation); Maggie Brooks-Carter (Scottish Massage Schools); Raymond Catchpole (Feng Shui Society); Bridget O'Connell (MIND); Jeremiah Solak (The Science Museum); Julie Doyle (The British Chiropractic Association).

The author would like to dedicate this book to her children, Jonathan, Philip and Charlotte.